Third Edition

Ethics, Jurisprudence, & Practice Management in Dental Hygiene

Vickie J. Kimbrough-Walls, RDH, MBA
Charla J. Lautar, RDH, PhD

Pearson

Boston   Columbus   Indianapolis   New York   San Francisco   Upper Saddle River
Amsterdam   Cape Town   Dubai   London   Madrid   Milan   Munich   Paris   Montreal   Toronto
Delhi   Mexico City   Sao Paulo   Sydney   Hong Kong   Seoul   Singapore   Taipei   Tokyo

Publisher: Julie Levin Alexander
Assistant to Publisher: Regina Bruno
Editor-in-Chief: Mark Cohen
Executive Editor: John Goucher
Assistant Editor: Nicole Ragonese
Media Editor: Amy Peltier
Media Project Manager: Lorena Cerisano
Production Manager: Kathleen Sleys
Creative Director: Jayne Conte
Cover Designer: Suzanne Behnke
Director of Marketing: David Gesell
Executive Marketing Manager: Katrin Beacom
Marketing Specialist: Michael Sirinides
Composition: Aptara®, Inc.
Printer/Binder: Edwards Brothers Malloy
Cover Printer: Lehigh/Phoenix Color Corp.
Cover Credits: Fotolia: Compass © Irochka

Notice:
The authors and the publisher of this volume have taken care that the information and technical recommendations contained herein are based on research and expert consultation and are accurate and compatible with the standards generally accepted at the time of publication. Nevertheless, as new information becomes available, changes in clinical and technical practices become necessary. The reader is advised to carefully consult manufacturers' instructions and information material for all supplies and equipment before use and to consult with a health care professional as necessary. This advice is especially important when using new supplies or equipment for clinical purposes. The authors and publisher disclaim all responsibility for any liability, loss, injury, or damage incurred as a consequence, directly or indirectly, of the use and application of any of the contents of this volume.

Library of Congress Cataloging-in-Publication Data

Kimbrough-Walls, Vickie J.
   Ethics, jurisprudence & practice management in dental hygiene / Vickie
J. Kimbrough-Walls, Charla J. Lautar.—3rd ed.
      p. ; cm.
   Other title: Ethics, jurisprudence, and practice management in dental hygiene
   Includes bibliographical references and index.
   ISBN-13: 978-0-13-139492-6
   ISBN-10: 0-13-139492-4
   1. Dental hygiene—Practice.   2. Dental ethics.   3. Dental
jurisprudence.   I. Lautar, Charla J., 1949-   II. Title.   III. Title:
Ethics, jurisprudence, and practice management in dental hygiene.
   [DNLM: 1. Practice Management, Dental—organization & administration.
2. Dental Hygienists. 3. Ethics, Dental. 4. Legislation, Dental. WU 77]
   RK60.5.K563 2012
   174'.96176—dc22   2010037346

10 9 8 7 6 5 4 3

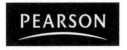

www.pearsonhighered.com

ISBN-10:   0-13-139492-4
ISBN-13: 978-0-13-139492-6

CONTENTS

PREFACE

The practice of dental hygiene continues to evolve in both scope of duties and changes in legislation. New workforce models are currently being offered for those interested in alternative settings and flexibility for providing oral health care to those with limited or no access to a dental office. Additionally, more health care providers are being sought in the profession of forensics in the event of catastrophes.

The information and examples in this book are designed to orient dental hygiene students to clinical practice and its many applications in an office setting. Although dental practices and dental hygiene procedures can be generalized, each office will be unique in its daily operations and policies. As public health is woven through the various roles of the dental hygienist, this book contains limited discussions regarding public health issues; however, it is not intended to replace the community health textbook you are presently using.

ORGANIZATION OF THE TEXT

Ethics, Jurisprudence, & Practice Management in Dental Hygiene is organized into 11 chapters and divided into two major sections: ethics and jurisprudence, and practice management as it applies to the dental hygienist as an employee and potential independent practitioner. The first two chapters introduce codes of ethics and discuss ethical principles, moral values, and how each influences society, individual, and the profession. Chapters 3 and 4 present informed consent and decision making as they relate to patients and the practioner, and Chapters 5 and 6 discuss legal information and social issues where the dental hygienist should be knowledgable, and as they may be applied to patient care.

The second half of the text will cover practice management. Chapters 7 and 8 introduce you to the dental practice and how it must operate as a small business. Chapter 9 is new and presents current information on workforce models such as the dental therapist and the registered dental hygienist in alternative practice. Chapters 10 and 11 provide information on interviewing, seeking your first dental hygiene position, and planning for a long-term career in your new profession.

At the end of the book are listed references, key terms in a glossary, and Internet resources. Throughout the book are boxes that highlight and condense information that was previously discussed. Follow-ups and critical-thinking questions integrate the chapter's content with the chapter's case study.

Chapter Format

Each chapter is consistent in its presentation of information and includes the following:

Objectives are statements designed to inform the student about the overall knowledge gained from chapter information.

Key Terms are listed at the beginning of each chapter and you will find them bolded and italicized in the text as you read through the chapter. They emphasize important concepts or major points of chapter content. These terms are also found at the end of the book in the glossary.

Case Studies The case studies present short scenarios that introduce and highlight chapter content. Some include a task or ask you to consider applying the chapter to the case in order to better understand how it applies to you as a dental hygiene professional.

Critical Thinking questions are found at the end of each chapter. These questions help you to insure your knowledge of the chapter content is correct, and some can be used for classroom discussion.

SPECIAL FEATURES

This third edition includes information regarding the practice of dental hygiene in Canada and internationally. Canadian dental hygienists are similar to American dental hygienists in many ways but differ in that the majority of them practice under self-regulation. In this global economy and transient society, it is important to be prepared for the opportunities of one's profession.

Also new to this edition is information on the new workforce models being offered and developed in the United States such as dental therapists, the registered dental hygienist in alternative practice, collaborative practice, and most recently, unsupervised practice in Maine. Aspects of practice management have expanded to include production goal setting, more business planning for dental hygiene, and identifying characteristics for leadership skills. You will find additional case studies located on MyHealthProfessionsKit along with many more resources designed to prepare you for entering the dental hygiene profession.

TEACHING AND LEARNING PACKAGE

Ethics, Jurisprudence, & Practice Management in Dental Hygiene has been written with the student in mind. Each chapter provides background information so that students without previous dental experience can better relate to topics in the text and apply them to clinical experiences they may have had during their dental hygiene education. The content provided in the text will enhance the development of professionalism students learn as they interact with peers and patients through a broad spectrum of topics for discussion and application to real situations.

For the Student

As a student, you will find the case studies in each chapter essential to better comprehension of the chapter content and how it applies to the practice of dental hygiene upon graduation. The MyHealthProfessionsKit includes more case studies related to ethical decision making along with Internet resources and business plan templates that may be required for assignments. For additional information please go to www.myhealthprofessionskit.com.

For the Instructor

Ethics, Jurisprudence, & Practice Management in Dental Hygiene now includes updated information on the new workforce models for oral health care professionals: dental therapists, advanced dental therapists, the Alaskan model (DHAT), and more. Additionally, new case studies are found in this edition and the previous case studies can be found on the MyHealthProfessionsKit website. This third edition has updated PowerPoint presentations that can be enhanced to customize your own lecture style and content, along with test bank questions to include on quizzes or tests. There is also a teaching tip component that offers suggestions for classroom activities and assignments. For additional information, please go to www. myhealthprofessionskit.com.

STUDY TIPS FOR STUDENTS

Many dental hygiene students use multiple methods for learning course content. The use of technology provides unlimited resources for gathering data and more examples to enhance student learning. The MyHealthProfessionsKit website provided for you with this text is one more way technology may assist in your overall understanding of the material and how it applies to the dental hygienist.

As you read and participate in the critical-thinking exercises, keep in mind that experiences will be unique. In this new millennium, the art and science of dental hygiene continue to progress and evolve. Consider the following as they apply to the content of each chapter:

✓ Supervision laws have been relaxed that allow for increase access to care and help eliminate disparities among diverse and underserved population groups.
✓ Strategies are being developed to increase cultural competencies and multidisciplinary collaboration as well as to increase the number of minorities in the oral health workforce.
✓ Dental hygienists are using more of their skills as oral health is becoming an important entity of general health.
✓ Dental hygienists are becoming more responsible for the regulation of their profession.

As a student, actively discuss dental situations you have previously experienced in your dental hygiene education. On becoming a registered or licensed dental hygienist, you are encouraged to actively participate in furthering the development of patient education and dental hygiene research as well as your own education. Reach out to communities that are not able to access dental care in a traditional setting and continually stay abreast of the link between periodontal disease and total body health, as patients see the dental hygienist as the oral health care specialist. The knowledge and relationships that build from networking with other professionals will be invaluable.

We hope that you find personal and professional satisfaction in your dental hygiene career and as a member of the dental hygiene profession. As dental hygienists move outside the isolated private dental office and globalism facilitates the exchange of information and culture, embrace dental hygiene wherever your future may be.

ACKNOWLEDGMENTS

To my sons, Kris, Lenny, and Rik—you continue to become my best friends and appreciate my pursuits in higher education, my mom Joanne, for her continuous pride in my achievements, and my, husband Mick—thank you for understanding my responsibilities and being patient as I juggle all these balls in the air.

I appreciate the many educators I have been in contact with during my career and respect the collaborative efforts to advance dental hygiene in all aspects of its potential. Special thanks to my fellow faculty at Truckee Meadows Community College for having open minds and the willingness to try new ideas that contribute to our positive learning environment and continued achievements.

Vickie J. Kimbrough-Walls, RDH, MBA

Thank you to Dr. Mohamed Elsamahi for his support and advice throughout the writing of the third edition. I would also like to thank those individuals and fellow dental hygienists who contributed case studies for this text and previous editions, including the Instructor's Manual, which are now on the website MyHealthProfessionsKit. In particular, I would like to recognize Teri McSherry for her case study in chapter four and to thank fellow dental hygiene educators Debbie Boyke and Judi Thomas for their prewriting encouragement with this edition.

Charla J. Lautar, RDH, PhD

REVIEWERS

Third Edition Reviewers

Marsha Bower, RDH, CDA, MA
Monroe Community College
Rochester, New York

Amy E. Cooper, RDH, BA
Tarrant County College
Hurst, Texas

Renee Cornett, RDH, MBA
Austin Community College
Austin, Texas

Laura Cunningham, MEd
University of Oklahoma
Oklahoma City, Oklahoma

Ann Curtis, RD, RDH, MS, CAS
University of Maine at Augusta
Bangor, Maine

Jacquelyn L. Fried, RDH, MS
University of Maryland Dental School
Baltimore, Maryland

Tracy Gift RDH, MS
Mohave Community College
Bullhead City, Arizona

Robin B. Matloff, RDH, BSDH, JD
Mount Ida College
Newton, Massachusetts

Shelly A. Purtell, RDH, MA
Broome Community College
Binghamton, New York

Salim Rayman, RDH, BS, MPA
Hostos Community College
Bronx, New York

Maribeth Stitt, RDH, MEd
Lone Star College—Kingwood
Kingwood, Texas

Sharon Struminger, RDH, MPS, MA
Farmingdale State College
Farmingdale, New York

Rebecca G. Tabor, RDH, MEd
Western Kentucky University
Bowling Green, Kentucky

Previous Edition Reviewers

Doni L Bird, RDH, MS
Santa Rosa Junior College
Santa Rosa, California

Ann Brunick, RDH, MS
University of South Dakota
Vermillion, South Dakota

Geraldine Hernandez, RDH
Miami Dade College
Miami, Florida

Sandra Horne, RDH, MHSA
University of Mississippi Medical Center
Jackson, Mississippi

Jacquelyn W. Johnson, RDH, MS
Tarrant County College—Northeast
Hurst, Texas

Bernice A. Mills, RDH, MS
University of New England
Portland, Maine

Nichole Oocumma, RDH, MA, CHES
Stark State College
North Canton, Ohio

Carolyn Ray, RDH, MEd
Texas Woman's University
Denton, Texas

David C. Reff, DDS
Apollo College
Boise, Idaho

Bonnie Tollinger, CDA
Boise State University
Boise, Idaho

W. Gail Barnes, RDH, PhD
Massachusetts College of Pharmacy
and Health Sciences
Boston, Massachusetts

Chris French Beatty, RDH, PhD
Texas Woman's University
Denton, Texas

Donna J. Stach, RDH, MEd
University of Colorado
Denver, Colorado

Barbara Paige, RDH, EdD
Cabrillo College
Aptos, California

Angelina E. Riccelli, RDH, MS
University of Pittsburgh
Pittsburgh, Pennsylvania

CHAPTER 1

Introduction to Moral Philosophy and Moral Reasoning

OBJECTIVES

After reading the material in this chapter, you will be able to

- Define the term *ethics.*
- Define the terms *deontology* (deontological approach) and *teleology* (teleological approach).
- Distinguish between the ethical theory of *utilitarianism* and *Kant's* ethical theory.
- Compare *rule* utilitarianism with *act* utilitarianism.
- Contrast a *right* with a *duty* and a *right* with a *privilege.*
- Discuss the role of *social justice* in determining ethical behavior.

KEY TERMS

Act utilitarian	Ethics	Rights
Consequentialist theory	Normative ethics	Rule utilitarian
Deontology	Prima facie	Teleology
Duty	Privilege	Virtue ethics

INTRODUCTION

Throughout our personal and professional lives, we make judgments and behave according to moral principles. These actions may be perceived as right or wrong based on their consequences, an individual's duties, and virtues or character traits. These perceptions have a profound effect on our view, as health care providers and as ordinary citizens, of access to health care and other social justice issues. This chapter serves as a knowledge foundation for decision making and actions in dental hygiene practice.

> ## Case Study
>
> After a conversation with your supervising employer dentist about universal health care, you tell her that covering every individual should be the aim. She argues against this proposition because this kind of health care coverage will lower the incomes of dentists and the entire office staff working with them.
>
> **As you read this chapter, consider the following:** Which ethical theory has guided you position?

ETHICAL THEORIES: DUTIES AND CONSEQUENCES

In health care and elsewhere, ethical behavior is the result of perceiving an action as either right or wrong. This perception is based on norms, duties, consequences, and character traits.

Ethics

The discipline of **ethics** consists of thoughts and ideas about morality. Ethics (or moral thinking) is concerned with studying human behavior, particularly toward other human beings, and the principles that can regulate it. Most ethical thinkers are philosophers, and philosophy differs from social sciences in its tendency to suggest or recommend standards, or norms, of behavior. For example, a sociologist may study the phenomenon of aggression, focusing on the causes of aggression and how some members of society become aggressive under certain circumstances. Similarly, a psychologist may explain why some people fail to develop normal empathic attitudes to others and become indifferent and insensitive to human suffering. A philosopher, on the other hand, would deal with aggression and insensitivity to suffering as violations of several moral values and would propose arguments to support the importance of peaceful and mutually respectful attitudes to human life and to other people.

Normative Ethics

The difference is that science, whether social or physical, is mainly descriptive, while moral philosophy is mainly normative. Science analyzes phenomena in depth and explains them. It may also predict future events on the basis of present observations. Ethical philosophy goes beyond studying phenomena at a descriptive level and proceeds to recommend desirable attitudes. Because desirable attitudes are commonly called *norms*, ethical thinking that purports to guide human behavior is called **normative ethics**.

Traditionally, the ethical studies that explore the nature of moral judgments and the structure of moral concepts are called *metaethics*. Metaethical studies investigate, for example, the meaning or the significance of what is right or wrong (good or evil) and whether moral judgments are objective or subjective (Honderich, 1995, p. 555). Normative ethics is the branch of metaethics that is concerned with moral recommendations about which acts are right and which are wrong. The study of normative ethics that is relevant to health care ethics can be divided into two major groups of theories: deontology and teleology. Virtue ethics is also an important normative position and will be discussed later in another section of this chapter.

DEONTOLOGY   The first normative ethical theory is **deontology**. Advocates of deontological ethics emphasize duties. For them, performing moral duties is not a matter of deliberation or negotiation. A **duty** is an obligation, an act that has to be done or ought to be done regardless of its consequences. In that way, deontological ethics shares with religions the concept of absolute obligation. A deontologist, for example, would expect people to tell the truth no matter what happens as a result. This is similar to the attitude of a religious person who never lies because lying is against the Ten Commandments. Ethical duties are derived from ethical principles and concepts. Some of these duties (e.g., truthfulness) are adopted by health care professions and stated in codes of professional ethics. Other duties (e.g., respect for private property) are incorporated into the legal system, while others (e.g., respect for personal privacy and helping the poor or elderly) are incorporated into social traditions and customs (Weinstein, 1993, p. 84). Purtilo (1999) defines three basic duties: absolute, prima facie, and conditional (p. 60). An absolute duty is binding under all circumstances. For example, the duty not to kill an innocent person is absolute because we know of no situation in which such killing would be permissible. It is important to notice here (or in that respect) that having to defend oneself against a non-innocent aggressor, which may result in killing in self-defense, is not a violation of deontology.

Prima facie duties differ in that they are determined by the present situation. The term *prima facie* means "at first glance," and a prima facie duty is a duty that is made obvious by the circumstances surrounding it. In dentistry, a scenario to illustrate this is treating the patient who is in pain before treating the patient who has come for a routine scheduled appointment. Treating the patient in pain seems to be the right decision even though it may upset the scheduled patient because of unexpected waiting.

A *conditional duty* is a commitment that comes into being after certain conditions are met. For instance, our society has a duty to support unemployed persons only after they try to learn new skills that may enable them to find jobs, or after it becomes obvious that they have no chance to find employment. Similarly, we have a duty to support medical research only after ensuring that it is well designed, feasible, and concerned with major health problems rather than with academic curiosities. Duties are further discussed in this chapter and in Chapter 2.

TELEOLOGY   Thus far, we have discussed the deontological group of theories. Let us examine the second group of normative theories, which is called *teleological* theories. The term **teleology** is derived from the Greek word for "end," or "goal." A teleologist will consider the consequences of telling the truth versus the consequences of lying and may find that lying is morally justified in a specific circumstance. This position, which is also called *consequentialism*, is based on the notion that what matters for morality is the result, or consequence, of an action. Telling a "little white lie" that will do more good than telling the truth counts, for teleologists, as a good action. For example, a teleologist would say that lying to a known killer about the hiding place of his potential victim is morally good. So the difference between deontologists and teleologists is that the former are concerned with the principle behind an action, while the latter are concerned with the results of an action.

ETHICAL THEORIES: A SURVEY OF MORAL THEORIES

In this section, three ethical theories will be discussed: utilitarianism, Kantian ethics, and virtue ethics. These theories provide a background or rationale for making moral judgments.

Utilitarianism

UTILITY AND CONSEQUENCES   The first utilitarians were the British philosophers Jeremy Bentham and John Stuart Mill, who lived in the nineteenth century. They argued that the aim of morality is attaining the greatest amount of utility for human beings and identified utility (or use-fulness) with happiness. Their theory, which became popular during much of the twentieth century in Britain and North America, is a **consequentialist theory**. Consequentialist (teleological) theories are based on the results of actions rather than on the nature of actions. For instance, if telling a lie can lead to saving an innocent life in a particular situation, it is morally good to tell a lie in that situation. That is, an action is morally right if it leads to desirable results and is wrong if it leads to undesirable results. Utilitarianism defines the "good consequence," or "desirable result," as the *maximal happiness* in the world (i.e., happiness for most people). According to utilitarianism, suffering is the ultimate evil and happiness the ultimate good, and the role of morality is to guide us to eliminate suffering and maximize happiness.

HAPPINESS   Utilitarianism does not recommend that every person pursue only what promotes his or her happiness. Instead, it recommends that all persons act in a way that leads to the least misery and the most happiness (including personal happiness) in the world. The utility principle recommends that we seek the "general" or "total" happiness in society rather than our own personal happiness. However, utilitarians do not ask us to ignore our own happiness but rather to view it as a part of total happiness. In that respect, utilitarianism adopts the principle of beneficence, which is discussed in Chapter 2. The beneficence principle requires one to do what is good for others without expecting a reward for doing so. Box 1-1 gives an example of utilitarianism.

BOX 1-1

Example

To understand utilitarianism, consider this example. A healthy man knows that his neighbor's daughter needs a kidney transplant to survive after a disease has destroyed both her kidneys. He volunteers to have his tissues tested for compatibility with the girl's tissues, and the result turns out to be positive. If he donates his kidney to save the girl's life, he exposes himself to a major surgical operation. He also knows that if he lives with only one kidney, there is a small chance of having a disease in that kidney in the future that may be severe enough to kill him. Donating his kidney would cost him at least some peace of mind. Should he accept this price (i.e., some anxiety about future health) and give the girl one of his kidneys? Utilitarians would encourage him to do so as long as he is unlikely to be significantly harmed. By saving her life, he makes her and her family and friends happy. He also makes people who advocate benevolent actions happy by giving a good example of benevolent behavior that may inspire others. The outcome of his action, then, would be more happiness in the world, and this agrees with the utility principle.

But utilitarians would not encourage a person who is likely to be harmed by a surgical operation to donate his kidney. As soon as the girl and her family realize that the benevolent man has exposed himself to a great danger, they would feel sorry rather than happy and thankful. At the same time, the man's own family and friends would be unhappy if he is harmed. In the end, his action would not add to the total happiness in the world and is therefore unethical on utilitarian grounds. So utilitarianism does not expect from any individual sacrifices that would not maximize happiness and minimize suffering for the greatest number of people.

When utilitarians discuss happiness, they do not mean any form of happiness. Happiness can be shallow, short lasting, significant, long lasting, hedonic (in the form of pleasurable feeling), or intellectual (e.g., enjoying an artwork). Short-term happiness is not the aim of utilitarianism. No utilitarian, for example, would encourage a student fond of sports to abandon school to satisfy the passion for sports or an art lover with limited resources to spend most of her income collecting paintings. It is also important to recognize that utilitarianism does not construe happiness merely as pleasure. Satisfaction in general, whether it derives from meeting one's basic needs, reading interesting novels, or helping the poor, would count as happiness for utilitarians. Another important point is that utilitarians regard reducing suffering (or decreasing unhappiness) equivalent to increasing happiness in the world. A dental hygienist who donates time to a public aid clinic thinking that the consequences will bring happiness to others is guided by the utility principle. If the dental hygienist who donates time to the public aid clinic instead of working for a salary is not able to provide for his or her children, then he or she is not following the utilitarian principle.

CATEGORIES OF UTILITARIANISM   There are two versions of utilitarianism: act utilitarianism and rule utilitarianism.

- An **act utilitarian** is concerned with individual acts. This person would assert that acting in a certain way (e.g., keeping promises) promotes general happiness, and for that reason, it is a good action.
- A **rule utilitarian**, on the other hand, is concerned more with the rule from which an action is derived. He or she would assert that the goodness of an action depends on whether it is justified by a rule that, if followed, can maximize happiness in the world.

There seems to be no substantial difference between the two positions. However, in some situations, rule utilitarianism can avoid problems that act utilitarianism cannot. As dental hygienists, we know that polishing teeth can damage tooth structure (Wilkins, 2009). Many patients feel that they have not received complete treatment unless the teeth are polished even though they are told about the disadvantages of polishing (patient may not have stains, polishing is contraindicated, no therapeutic reason). In order to provide happiness to the patient, the dental hygienist gives the illusion of polishing by sweeping the rubber cup over the surfaces of the teeth with minimal or no pressure. The patient feels the act of polishing and tastes the polishing agent.

It is difficult to describe a deceptive act as morally good, yet a rule utilitarian would not agree that the dental hygienist's action was good because adopting the rule that deceiving people in order to please them would not maximize happiness. Rational people would feel unhappy and even angry if they knew that they were deceived in order to be pleased. It would be wrong to suggest to a patient that a procedure was done when in fact it was not.

RELEVANCY OF UTILITARIANISM   Is utilitarianism relevant to health care ethics? Yes, because this theory is concerned with reducing suffering, which is one of the main duties of health care providers. Moreover, utilitarianism contributes significantly to the discussion of the problem of fair distribution of health care resources.

Case Study Follow-up #1

In the chapter's case study, the dental hygienist is taking the position of a utilitarian or using the utilitarianism ethical theory to defend universal health care. The dental hygienist perceives that universal health care will bring happiness to most people.

Kantian Ethics

MORALLY RIGHT ACT OR A DUTY According to Immanuel Kant, the eighteenth-century German philosopher, certain acts are morally right because they are intrinsically right regardless of their consequences or results. Consequences, he asserts, should not matter when the moral value of an action is assessed. Kant even argues that consequences are relevant to practical matters, not to ethics. In the practical realm, one has to ask will this action can lead to good results and act accordingly. For example, a student may decide to study engineering because engineers have good careers. Such a decision is based on consequential (teleological) considerations: studying engineering qualifies one to enter a stable and rewarding career. When that student decided to be an engineer to enjoy the benefits that result from this decision, he or she was making a consequentialist but purely practical decision. But the situation is different in the moral realm.

In the moral field, there are acts that must be done whether or not they lead to desirable or undesirable results. Therefore, these acts are moral duties, Kant asserts. These acts lose moral worth when they are done to attain an aim. For example, if you do not tell lies because you want to impress people and get their support or votes, you are either acting practically (from practical motives) or immorally (by trying to exploit ethical principles for material gain). However, if you do not tell lies because you believe that lying is morally wrong, you are acting morally. In other words, you are performing a moral duty. Because Kant's ethics is concerned with duties and reduces moral principles to duties, it was called *deontological* (from the Greek *deon*, meaning "obligation").

MORAL PRINCIPLES Kant opposed deriving moral principles from accidental events and contingencies because that could lead to formulating contradictory principles. Suppose that a freedom fighter in Poland during World War II gave the Nazi officers who were interrogating him false information about the identities of his partners. By doing that, he saved their lives and served a good cause. But can we derive from that circumstance a principle that justifies telling lies when it is convenient to do so? Kant's answer is an unequivocal no. For him, ethical principles cannot be subjected to negotiation, nor should they be modified to adapt to new situations when it appears useful to modify them. It is wrong, he believes, to modify one's commitment to truth telling in light of the present circumstances. Moral principles, Kant insists, should be based on solid foundations then followed with total disregard for the context. If we believe that truth telling is good, we must always tell the truth even if that leads to great harm in a particular context. Thus, the Polish freedom fighter did not act according to sound moral principles when he lied to the Nazis, in Kant's opinion.

Kant acknowledged that it is sometimes harmful to follow moral principles faithfully. He knew very well that, at least in exceptional cases, we might do better by violating moral principles. But he argued that repeated violations could send a harmful message to people. Violations (or variations) may suggest that one is encouraged to violate moral principles when it seems useful to do so. Kant believed interpreting moral principles in a relative way permits us to lie today and then tell the truth tomorrow and opens the door for moral confusion and chaos. Consequently, moral principles should be absolute (unmodifiable). So the main issue in Kantian ethics is that there are *categorical* (absolute) imperatives (duties) that are inescapable. They can be inferred by reason and should be generalized.

MORAL DUTY Kant's contention that duties are categorical is disputable. However, his view that we must treat all people as ends in themselves, not as means, is widely respected. How does he argue for that principle? According to Kant, every human being is a rational person. And rational persons appreciate and value their rationality. As a result, they would not accept being used or treated as means. Their self-respect and respect for the value of rationality would not allow that. It follows that no person should accept being treated as a means to other ends and that every person ought to be treated as an end in himself or herself. This principle is highly esteemed in ethics and in health care ethics in particular. As will be seen later, it follows from this principle that people should not be treated as objects, and as a result, their well-being (and health) should not be treated as a commodity. Using the previous example, the dental hygienist who donates time to a public aid clinic because it is a *moral* duty—even if this means losing salary, sacrificing leisure time, or denying his or her children small pleasures—to help the disadvantaged is guided by deontological or Kantian principle.

Case Study Follow-up #2

In the chapter's case study, what is the moral duty of the dentist?

Virtue Ethics

CHARACTER TRAITS **Virtue ethics** places emphasis on character traits of individuals and was advocated by the early philosophers such as Socrates, Plato, and Aristotle. According to them, virtue is the basis of morality. They regarded persons of excellent character as moral persons. That is, a virtuous person is essentially a person who acts morally. The virtue approach to ethics demands that every person think and act in the best way possible for a given situation (Ozar & Sokol, 1994, p. 4). For example, a virtuous person would advocate fairness and equal respect for people's interests when a conflict between individuals arises and requires mediation or arbitration. He or she would also recommend kindness to animals, honesty in financial dealings, and truth telling. In other words, virtuous people are disposed to think and act morally. This disposition (or readiness to act in a certain way) is taken by the proponents of virtue ethics as the guide to moral judgments.

Advocates of virtue ethics expect and require every person to act like a virtuous person. By doing so, they act in a morally good way. This shows that virtue ethics relies on the moral inclination of people with excellent personal qualities to identify the morally right and wrong. Obviously, this approach differs from other systems or theories of metaethics (e.g., deontology and teleology) that rely on rules, principles, consequences, or goals. That is, virtue ethics tells us to act the way a virtuous person would act in a similar situation, while other theories tell us to act according to the principle or rule that suits the situation. Such a principle or rule may derive from Kantian or utilitarian theories, for example. Box 1-2 reviews the types of normative ethics.

Historically, the ancient virtue ethics emphasized the cardinal virtues of temperance, justice, courage, and wisdom. In the Middle Ages, Christianity added the theological virtues of faith, hope, and charity. Many feel that a person cannot possess one virtue without the other and that all virtues are interrelated or interdependent. In other words, a person who is courageous and truthful would also be fair and benevolent. But virtue ethics, which was ignored in modern times, is no longer dead. There are contemporary philosophers who think that a focus on virtue, not on abstract principles, can form the basis for morality (Honderich, 1995, p. 901).

BOX 1-2

Types of Normative Ethics

Teleology: type of ethics that emphasizes consequences

Deontology: type of ethics that emphasizes duties

Virtue ethics: type of ethics that emphasizes character traits

SOCIAL PHILOSOPHY

Social philosophy deals with issues like justice, rights, and equality. Problems in medical ethics that belong to the area of social philosophy include, among other things, equal access to health care resources and patients' rights.

Utilitarianism and Justice

SOCIAL JUSTICE   Utilitarianism is meant to be a social philosophy as well as a general theory of normative ethics. The utilitarian view of justice is considered the most important component in the social aspect of utilitarianism. Utilitarians understand social justice as a means to happiness. They argue that satisfying basic needs leads to more happiness than does enjoying luxuries. A nice weekend in Hawaii would make any person feel happy. But there are degrees of happiness. Compare the happiness that a vacationing person in Hawaii would experience with the happiness that a starving, chilled person would experience when fed and warmed. The utilitarians are warranted in asserting that satisfying essential needs creates greater pleasure than satisfying less basic needs. Moreover, lacking basic needs, such as adequate food and shelter, is apt to create suffering, while giving up some luxuries is unlikely to produce significant discomfort.

Consequently, taking some resources from people who have already satisfied all their basic needs and giving them to those whose basic needs are not satisfied would increase the amount of total happiness in the world. And this is the declared aim of utilitarianism. So justice, as conceived by utilitarians, is a process that is meant to maximize happiness and reduce suffering. It is not an end in itself, though.

HEALTH CARE IMPLICATIONS   The implications of social justice for health care ethics are great. A society in which the majority of people are unable to obtain health care cannot be called a happy society. Sickness produces suffering and undermines happiness; and whenever the number of sick or improperly treated people in a society is large, happiness in this society is limited. It follows that making health care resources available for all or most members of society is essential for keeping the level of happiness in that society sufficiently high. This is how utilitarians justify the necessity of distributing health care resources (or goods) fairly among all people. It is important to notice that utilitariansim calls not for complete equality but rather for the extent of equality that keeps most people healthy and free of suffering.

Liberalism and Rights

RIGHTS   Social philosophy talked about duties but not rights until John Locke, the 18th-century British philosopher, emphasized the concept of natural rights. Locke's aim was to fight the tyranny of European governments and the vulnerability of the ordinary citizen to the unrestricted power of governments. He argued that human beings are born with **rights** attached to them by nature, including the right to freedom (autonomy), life, property ownership, and free expression. The elite were the only people granted these rights at that time. Even the elite, other than the monarchs, were not allowed free expression in most circumstances. Citizens in Locke's time were granted limited rights through government decrees and statutes. These did not include the right to free speech or the pursuit of personal happiness.

In the Constitution of the United States, Americans were granted the right to life, liberty, and the pursuit of happiness. Additional rights, such as freedom of speech and bearing arms, were given later in the U.S. Bill of Rights. The notion of rights has advanced social and political philosophies to a large extent. In fact, the notions of human rights, equal civil rights, and freedom from oppression that dominated the twentieth century's movements of social and political reform were inspired by liberalism. Furthermore, the political aspect of liberalism is behind most of the principles of international law.

DUTY   A right is defined as a valid claim. If a person is entitled to voting privileges and there are no sound legal reasons for denying this entitlement, he or she has a right (valid claim) to vote. This right allows him or her to expect other members of society not to interfere with his or her going to the polls and casting a vote. Rights, then, protect one's interests by imposing corresponding duties on other people to respect the interests of a right holder. In other words, every right has a corresponding duty on the part of other society members. Without such duty, exercising a right would be difficult. For example, your right to privacy cannot be exercised if your society does not consider it a duty to protect you from intruders. This is why no citizen in the former Soviet Union had a right to free speech: Citizens had no duty to help any person to express his or her opinions.

Three Facts about Rights

There are three important points about rights.

RIGHTS ARE NOT PRIVILEGES   There are three important points about rights. First, rights differ from ordinary freedoms (privileges). For example, every person is entitled to play chess or to go to music concerts. But no person should expect others to help him or her play chess or go to concerts because our society does not impose on us a duty to help other people enjoy freedoms. Yet every person expects others to help protect his or her property or privacy (either directly or by supporting the institutions that enforce law and order in society).

MORAL AND LEGAL RIGHTS   Second, there are moral rights and legal rights. Moral rights include the right to life, autonomy, and equality before the law. A moral right is a valid claim that is based on moral (ethical) reasons. For example, the right to life is based on the ethical principle that killing is wrong, and the right to autonomy is based on the principle that it is morally wrong to control other individuals. Although many moral rights are protected by law in most societies, some are not, so not every moral right is a legal right. Until the nineteenth century, for instance, slavery was legal in the United States. The moral right to autonomy was not considered a legal right at that time.

Some legal rights may not be moral rights. For example, firing workers without significant compensation and when there is no economic need for reducing the workforce is a legal right for employers in the United States but not in Germany or Sweden. Germans and Swedes, among others, think that this right is based on an unfair principle that ignores the well-being of workers. For an ethicist, the right of an employer to dismiss workers arbitrarily may seem difficult to accept on moral grounds although it is allowed by law.

RIGHTS ARE NOT ABSOLUTE   They can be revoked or suspended. For example, a criminal is deprived of his right to autonomy when he is kept in jail. Similarly, the right to free speech is restricted by the rights of other people not to be defamed or slandered. It is true that people have the right to express their opinions, but it is also true that they should not misuse their rights and insult or humiliate others in the process.

Is liberalism relevant to health care ethics? It enables medical ethics to utilize the concept of patients' rights and providers' corresponding duties to such rights. Without the concept of moral rights, which Locke called *natural rights*, it would be difficult to explore areas like privacy, confidentiality, informed consent, and paternalism. That will be seen more clearly in following chapters.

A right must not be confused with a **privilege**. As stated previously, a right is guaranteed for all persons. But privileges are not guaranteed (though not denied) for any person. No individual is entitled to claim the privilege of owning an expensive car or obtaining a license to practice dental hygiene. These privileges must be earned by effort and hard work. They are not guaranteed to whoever wants them. If a person wants to practice dental hygiene, he or she has to meet certain conditions required for licensure. Compare that with the right to life, for example. The right to life cannot be withheld, is not earned, and is guaranteed for all. Box 1-3 names three characteristics of rights.

CONTROVERSIES IN THE UNITED STATES   Controversies have arisen in the United States as to whether health care (including dental hygiene care) is a right for all residents or a privilege for those who can afford it through personal wealth or the ability to pay for insurance. And, if health care is ever guaranteed for all citizens, which benefits and procedures would be granted to every person who needs them? Would every treatment modality, regardless of its cost, be made available to all citizens who would benefit from them? Another controversy is education. Should postsecondary education be a privilege only for those who can afford the tuition? These are just a few examples that help distinguish privilege from right.

BOX 1-3

Characteristics of Rights

- For every right there is a corresponding duty.
- A right is guaranteed while a privilege is earned.
- A right can be taken away.

Rawls's Theory of Justice

John Rawls is a contemporary American philosopher whose main concern has been social justice. He proposed a theory in the early 1970s that characterizes social justice as a fair deal that members of society negotiate and abide by (Rawls, 1971).

JUSTICE AS AN END IN ITSELF   Contrary to the utilitarian view of justice as a means for happiness, Rawls asserts that justice is an end in itself. It is a situation that rational members of society desire and aspire to attain. Therefore, its principles cannot be arbitrary. These principles should be carefully sought and formulated. Meanwhile, the principles of justice cannot be reached by speculation that fails to consider the real wants and needs of people in society. If philosophers introduce principles of justice that are theoretically elegant and admirable but practically unrealizable or unacceptable to the average person, these principles will never work.

AGREEING ON WHAT IS JUST   Rawls's idea is that people do not need a profound thinker to advise them about justice. Rather, they need to reach an agreement among themselves, based on rational debate, that they accept and enact. People need to think impartially to reach a lasting agreement. Our experience with modern science tells us that scientists agree easily on the same conclusions and interpretations of data because they think impartially. Practitioners of science, when they strictly follow the scientific method, can be impartial. But impartiality is more difficult to achieve in daily life, where various kinds of biased attitudes influence people.

Yet Rawls finds a way out. He believes that people will be impartial if they are ignorant about their personal status, economic situation, and social standing. The reason is that people will not be biased to a group, profession, or class if they have no idea about where they stand. Imagine that you do not know whether you will be a professional, a merchant, a skilled laborer, or a manual worker. Would you take sides with those who demand equal tax cuts for every citizen so that the rich do not pay more than the poor? Or with those who advocate raising the minimum wage? Perhaps you would be rather neutral on both issues. But a low-income worker would typically side with the latter issue, while an owner of a corporation would side with the former. This seems natural because people tend to favor the proposals and plans that serve their own interests. This assumption that people act from self-interest underlies Rawls's theory.

VEIL OF IGNORANCE   Rawls calls the situation in which people can be impartial the *original position*. In this imaginary situation, people would discuss justice with (to speak metaphorically) a veil of ignorance in front of their eyes. Only in this situation, Rawls believes, could people think without preconceived biases and therefore reach reasonable agreements. His line of reasoning is that people think, argue, and act from self-interest. If someone knew that he or she would be a nuclear physicist, that person would believe that it is just to reward people with intellectual abilities. If the same person knew that he or she would be a factory worker, he or she would think that people should be rewarded according to the physical effort they expend to produce goods. However, if people were in the original position, they would agree on a system of principles that causes the least harm to any of them if they turn out to be in the least privileged class or group.

Rawls supposes (with good reasons) that in the original position, people would agree on principles that promote mutual self-interest and that they would not agree except on principles that further the interests of them all. Thus, self-interest in combination with rational thinking would impose a cautious attitude. Rational, self-interested people would not take risks; they would be careful. They would not assume that they might eventually be in the elite class, so in order to avoid harming themselves if they happen to be in a lower position, they would not choose principles that favor the top class. Rawls assumes that ignorance about one's future position would suppress the gambling, irrational attitude in people and would motivate them to think cautiously. In other words, they would be guided primarily by risk aversion.

BASIC LIBERTIES   Self-interest, moreover, would guide people to insist on equal basic liberties for all. Such liberties include free speech, autonomy, equal opportunities, and similar essential freedoms. Not many people, in Rawls's opinion, would be willing to sacrifice these badly needed liberties. Self-interest would also direct them to prefer abundance with some degree of inequality to equality with scarcity because satisfying basic needs comes before the need for fairness, at least for most people. As Rawls sees it, any person would prefer to have a big piece of a large pie that is cut into unequal but sizable pieces rather than a tiny piece of a smaller pie that is cut into exactly equal pieces (so that every person gets an equal share). That is, Rawls thinks that every reasonable person would say, "I want to eat enough, no matter how much the other guy is eating." What Rawls wants to conclude here is that justice cannot be absolute and that the demand for justice is restricted by other factors, particularly by the need for abundance.

It follows that if the motivation to work productively (which is essential for affluence) requires inequality (which will result from rewarding productive more than nonproductive people), it would be reasonable to allow the least possible degree of inequality required for increasing productivity. Based on this situation, people will conclude that justice can be established on two basic principles, commonly called Rawls's two principles of justice.

RAWLS'S TWO PRINCIPLES OF JUSTICE   The first principle says that each person has an equal right to the most extensive scheme of equal basic liberties that a society can afford. These liberties should be guaranteed for each person to the extent that they do not undermine the liberties of others. That is, no person can have a degree of liberty that, for being too much, decreases the amounts of liberties available to others (and consequently leads to inequality).

The second principle says that social and economic goods may be distributed unequally under two conditions. First, these inequalities should work for the benefit of the least advantaged. Second, they should be made open to fair competition in which all members of society can participate. All precautions must be taken to ensure that any person can fairly compete for advantaged positions. That is, these privileged positions must be given only to those who deserve them, not to members of an elite or favored class. Box 1-4 summarizes the two principles of justice.

BOX 1-4

Two Principles of Justice

- Each person has equal right to liberties as long as it does not mean that others have lesser unequal liberties.
- Social and economic goods may be unequal if (a) the inequalities work for the benefit of the least advantaged, and (b) there is open and fair competition for all to participate.

Why should the least advantaged be favored? This is an important question that poses itself at this point. Rawls's answer is that inequality is not a prize given to the gifted to express our admiration. It is a "carrot" to tempt the gifted to do their best for others. This is not an exploitation of the gifted, though. A gifted person may argue that hard work, not merely talent, earned him or her success. However, the motivation to work hard is determined by a personal quality that is derived from genes. What comes from nature is a resource, like water and minerals, and resources are liable to fair distribution. Unequal income, then, is not naturally deserved by the gifted but was granted them in a deal that was negotiated in the original, hypothetical position. Less gifted people chose to allow for such a privilege (which they could have chosen not to grant to the gifted) in return for a commitment by the gifted to pay back.

Rawls would, for example, say, "If you are an excellent entrepreneur while I am an ordinary person, I still have some right to your achievements because your intelligence is an asset like other natural resources. If your talent does not work for my advantage, you have done injustice to me because your talent (or resources like oil wells or rivers) should be used for everyone's benefit." So, according to Rawls's theory, the talented should realize that they have already entered an agreement in the original position to work first for the least advantaged. If they change their minds after becoming privileged, they should be reminded of their initial judgment and agreement, which was made when impartiality was possible (i.e., under the veil of ignorance).

Applying Rawls's Theory to Health Care Problems

How does this theory fit into the problems addressed by health care ethics? Remember that health care goods are limited, while the needs for them are immense. That is, there is a relative but significant scarcity of health care resources. These resources need to be distributed carefully. Should we allow the rich to have the best resources for themselves because they can afford to pay for them? Utilitarians disagree because favoring the rich or any particular section of society limits the general happiness to this section alone and lets the suffering of other sections grow. The ultimate result is a reduction in the total happiness in society, which is morally undesirable.

However, Rawls rejects tying justice to happiness. Yet he reaches the same utilitarian conclusion: Health care resources should be distributed fairly among all members of society. How does he justify this answer? Recall the original position. If people are in that position, which is conducive to impartiality, they will choose the arrangement that exposes them to the least risk. Since none of them knows whether he will be healthy or ill or able to pay medical bills or even buy necessary medications, he will choose a system that makes the most privileged responsible to work for improving the situation of the least advantaged.

EQUAL ACCESS TO BASIC HEALTH CARE   Reflect on the conclusions of utilitarianism and Rawls's theory. Both favor an arrangement that ensures that all—or at least most people—get equal access to basic health care services (e.g., emergency care and immunizations) and almost equal access to every other form of essential health care service. Utilitarians want that arrangement to increase the happiness in the world, and Rawls wants it because it agrees with people's attitudes and inclinations, at least when they think impartially. A system of national health insurance would be ideal for both philosophies, although any system that guarantees affordable care for every member of society would be acceptable to them.

Health care can be viewed as an economic good. Concerns regarding the equitable access to health care or health services are addressed with two theories: market justice and social justice. Shi and Singh (2004) provide the following comparison: Market justice views health care as an economic good, based on demand and one's ability to pay and as an economic reward. Thus, each individual is responsible for his or her own health. In addition, in market justice, benefits are based on the purchasing power of every individual. Social justice, on the other hand, views health as a social resource and a basic right. According to social justice, one's ability to pay is not a condition for receiving medical care, and the government is involved in health service delivery. So this view considers health care a collective (public) good (p. 59).

PRACTICAL RESTRICTIONS   Ideally, every person should have access to any form of health care that he or she needs. But the scarcity of resources imposes practical restrictions on distributing health care services and necessitates drawing a distinction, however arbitrary, between "badly needed" and "less urgently needed" services. Unfortunately, not all dental care or preventive dental hygiene care is considered "needed" health care in terms of insurance or government assistance programs (see Chapter 6). Let us hope that future advances in technology succeed in reducing the cost of health care.

Case Study Follow-up #3

Do you think health care is a right or a privilege? If a right, what is your duty?

Summary

The discipline of ethics consists of thoughts and ideas about morality. The study of normative ethics can be divided into two major groups of theories: deontology and teleology (consequentialism). Deontological theories (Kant's ethics) emphasize duties, while teleological theories emphasize consequences of actions. Utilitarianism is a teleological theory concerned with attaining the greatest amount of utility, usefulness, or happiness. Social philosophy is concerned mainly with rights of people and social justice. A right is a valid claim and is ensured for all people. A privilege, by contrast, is not guaranteed and must be attained by personal effort or optional help from people who want to provide such help. Although no person is obligated to help others attain a privilege, there is no moral rule that forbids volunteering to help someone to gain a privilege in a way that does not harm others. Utilitarians view social justice as a means to happiness, and for this reason, they pursue justice. Because utilitarianism considers justice a moral goal, it recommends that society allocate goods and services, such as health care resources, in a fair way.

Critical Thinking

1. How is the study of *ethics* different from other disciplines (or courses) you have previously studied?
2. Compare the term *deontology* with the term *teleology.*
3. What is the major difference between a *rule* utilitarian and an *act* utilitarian?
4. According to utilitarians, what is the role of the utility or the consequences of an action?
5. Give an example of (a) a *right*, (b) a *duty*, and (c) a *privilege*.
6. Explain how John Rawls's theory of justice is a theory of social justice.

7. Divide into groups. Relate to one another situations in which decisions had to be made. Classify the decisions based on the basis of the ethical theories or approaches. Present these findings to the class. Does the class agree with your classifications?

8. Design a case study or scenario that would involve a decision that a dental hygienist may have to make regarding patient care or a public health need. Select an ethical theory. Defend the decision using the selected ethical theory.

9. In pairs, role-play the dentist and the dental hygienist as described in this chapter's case study.

10. Hold a debate in class: Is health care a right or a privilege?

CHAPTER 2

Core Values and Additional Ethical Principles

OBJECTIVES

After reading the material in this chapter, you will be able to

- Identify the core values found in the Code of Ethics of the American Dental Hygienists' Association, the five main principles articulated in the Code of Ethics of the Canadian Dental Hygienists Association, and the two values embedded in the Code of Ethics of the International Federation of Dental Hygienists.

- Compare other codes of ethics found in the dental hygiene profession at the local, state, provincial, and national levels.

- Define the terms *autonomy, confidentiality, societal trust, nonmaleficence, beneficence, justice, veracity, fidelity, paternalism,* and *utility.*

KEY TERMS

Autonomy	HIPAA	Paternalism
Beneficence	Justice	Trust
Confidentiality	Nonmaleficence	Utility
Fidelity	Parentalism	Veracity

INTRODUCTION

Decisions and actions of health care providers are guided by ethical principles and core values. These core values are based on the Hippocratic oath and similar codes. They have evolved through the years as professions formulate their individual codes of ethics. The importance of a code of ethics in the practice of dental hygiene is illustrated in the curriculum document *Competencies for Entry into the Profession of Dental Hygiene.* The first core competency for all the roles of the dental hygienist: Apply a professional code of ethics in all endeavors (American Dental Education Association, 2003; www.adea.org)

This chapter will focus on the core values and additional ethical principles found in professional codes of ethics. Examples of how these principles can determine actions taken are provided to demonstrate the application of these principles in dental hygiene practice and other situations. Health information is also protected through legislation such as the Health Insurance Portability and Accountability Act (HIPAA).

Case Study

During a routine dental hygiene recall appointment for a 15-year-old female patient, you notice that she has plaque around the mandibular first premolar areas. These two teeth are rotated and in linguoversion. The patient has spoken to you about her concern about the unappealing appearance of her "lower" teeth and what can be done to make her smile more flattering. Additionally, she states that she finds these two areas very difficult to floss and to brush.

Both you and the dentist recommend to her and to her parents the possibility of orthodontic treatment for this area. The family has insurance coverage and is faithful about keeping recall appointments and other treatment needs such as sealants and restorations. However, the father is reluctant to obtain information regarding an orthodontic referral. The father protests and refuses to discuss the treatment, citing his spiritual belief that prohibits "changing creation" and "science's interference with Mother Nature."

As you read this chapter, consider the following: What ethical principles does the dental hygienist need to consider when developing a treatment plan for this patient?

CORE VALUES

Core values are selected ethical principles that are considered central to a particular code of ethics. In the Code of Ethics of the American Dental Hygienists' Association (ADHA), seven core values are identified: autonomy, confidentiality, societal trust, nonmaleficence, beneficence, justice, and veracity (www.adha.org). These are listed in Box 2-1. Similarly, the Code of Ethics of the Canadian Dental Hygienists Association (CDHA) names five main principles: beneficence, autonomy, privacy and confidentiality, accountability, and professionalism (www.cdha.ca). Likewise, the Code of Ethics of the International Federation of Dental Hygienists (IFDH) states two values: integrity and respect which includes honesty, respect for individual choices, and patient confidentiality (www.ifdh.org). Additionally information can be found at these websites.

The *ADEA Statement on Professionalism in Dental Education,* including dental hygiene education, identifies six values: competency, fairness, integrity, responsibility, respect, and service-mindedness (ADEA, 2009; www.adea.org). These values were adapted from Codes of Ethics of the American Dental Association, the American Dental Hygienists' Association, and the American Student Dental Association. Furthermore, application of this definition of professionalism is made regarding the behavior of students, faculty, researchers, and administrators especially as they oversee educational institutions. Thus, ethics and professionalism do interact.

BOX 2-1

Core Values of the ADHA Code of Ethics

Autonomy	To guarantee self-determination of the patient
Confidentiality	To hold in confidence or secret information entrusted by the patient
Societal Trust	To ensure the trust that patients and society have in dental hygienists
Nonmaleficence	To do no harm to the patient
Beneficence	To benefit the patient
Justice	To be fair to the patient; fairness; treat all patients equally
Veracity	To tell the truth; not to lie to the patient

Autonomy

The first core value is **autonomy**. Autonomy is *self-determination*. An autonomous person controls his or her own actions, behavior, and inner life (i.e., plans, goals, convictions, and beliefs). He or she also decides which values to advocate, which faith to adhere to, and which lifestyle to adopt.

As seen in Chapter 1, the Kantian principle of respect for persons implies that every individual should be valued and appreciated. It follows that the preferences of every person should be respected by fellow human beings. This is how the Kantian principle substantiates the concept of autonomy. The right to autonomy is among the fundamental rights emphasized by libertarian philosophers and proponents of human rights. Although the right to autonomy began as a moral right, that is, a right that morality calls for, it soon became an essential component of our legal rights.

Individuals should be able to decide for themselves what actions they will undertake even if these seem foolish to others. There are limits to autonomy. People are free to behave as they choose only as long as they do not harm others. Indeed, harm is the main restriction on autonomy. Fortunately, we can all be autonomous without harming each other because it is easy for rational persons to consider the interests of other persons and to act in a way that preserves them.

INFORMED CONSENT   What are the implications of autonomy for health care? If competent adults are granted the right to autonomy, they should be permitted to accept or refuse any actions that affect their lives. Consequently, competent patients (and guardians or parents of incompetent patients) should be allowed to accept or refuse treatment. Some patients have limited knowledge of health-related issues and therefore cannot decide on a proposed treatment unless they are informed about its effectiveness, cost, likelihood of success, side effects, and so on. As a result, it is the right of a patient to have adequate information about an action, such as an operation, that will affect his or her life. With this information, the person can agree to a treatment plan or refuse it. This is precisely how the notion of informed consent, discussed in the next chapter, is derived from the right to autonomy.

The ADHA Code of Ethics emphasizes the core value of individual autonomy and the rights that follow from it: "People have the right to be treated with respect. They have the right to informed consent prior to treatment, and they have the right to full disclosure of all relevant information so that they can make informed choices about their care" (American Dental Hygienists' Association, 1999, p. 17). Autonomy is also a main principle in the CDHA Code of Ethics, which highlights the right of patients to make their own choices (Canadian Dental Hygienists Association, 2002). Also, the IFDH Code of Ethics, outlines respect for persons and personal dignity, respect for individual choices to accept or decline services, and respect for human rights, values, customs, and spiritual beliefs (International Federation of Dental Hygienists, 2003).

Case Study Follow-up #1

In this chapter's case study, what are the restrictions on autonomy for the 15-year-old patient?

Confidentiality

The core value **confidentiality** is the avoidance of revealing any personal information about the patient. Personal information may be sensitive or even embarrassing, and failure to keep it within proper bounds can harm the patient in various ways. The practice of keeping private information about patients confidential should extend to all kinds of personal information, not just shameful or embarrassing information.

PROMISE   Confidentiality differs from privacy in that confidentiality involves a promise from a trusted person. If a person entrusts a friend not to publicize personal information, the friend implicitly promises to keep the information confidential. Similarly, patients giving their providers personal information about themselves assume that the providers are implicitly promising confidentiality (further discussion of confidentiality and privacy is found at www.cdha.org). Keeping a promise is a moral duty that every ethical theory emphasizes, so it would be unethical of providers to reveal any personal information relevant to their patients. Confidentiality is also a legal duty of health care providers and a patient's right (see Chapter 5).

It is true that patients who voluntarily give personal information to their providers are, in effect, giving up their right to privacy. The act of sharing information itself implies declining the right to privacy. But the right to privacy also includes the right to determine what will be shared with whom. Consequently, individuals declining their right to privacy by sharing personal information with providers do not lose their right to determine whether any other individual can have access to this information. Thus, the provider cannot pass personal information to any party without permission from the patient.

DISCLOSING INFORMATION   Confidentiality may be breached if there is a moral justification for disclosure or if the patient requests or consents to the disclosure. The Code of Ethics of the IFDH states: "The dental hygienist holds personal information confidential and uses professional reasoned judgment in sharing this information (IFDH, 2003; www.idhf.org). For example, one may disclose confidential information in certain cases to another health care provider if the information is relevant to helping the patient. Circumstances that allow for disclosing confidential information are found in Box 2-2.

BOX 2-2

Disclosing Confidential Information

1. In an emergency
2. To protect third parties
3. When required by law (e.g., sexually transmitted disease or child or elderly abuse) or policy of the practice environment (e.g., quality assurance)
4. When requesting commitment or hospitalization of a mentally ill patient
5. To guardian or substitute decision maker of incompetent patient

(Canadian Dental Hygienists Association, 2002; Gutheil & Appelbaum, 1982, 2000; Purtilo, 1999, p. 154)

A hypothetical example for an emergency in dental hygiene practice would be the following. A patient experiences chest pain in the dental chair, and you call for an ambulance. You remember that the patient told you that he abuses cocaine, and you have documented this in the medical history. Knowing that cocaine can induce severe, potentially fatal heart disease, you reveal to the paramedics on their arrival the information about your patient's substance abuse. Normally, no information from a patient's health history can be relayed to another provider without the patient signing a release form.

In this case, however, the information you give the paramedics will help in the diagnosis and treatment of the present chest pain and potential heart problem. Breach of confidentiality may occasionally be necessary to protect a third party. For example, a patient has more severe attrition on his teeth than on his last visit. He states that he grinds his teeth more since his divorce because he is still angry with his wife. He tells you that he will one day kill his wife for what she has done to him. Here you have an obligation to protect her by contacting her or the police because you know that threats made by emotionally upset people can be serious.

PROTECTION OF HEALTH INFORMATION   Even as early as 1948, the United Nations in the Universal Declaration of Human Rights recognized the need for confidentiality in Article 12: "No one shall be subjected to arbitrary interference with his privacy, family, home or correspondence, nor to attacks upon his honour [honor] and reputation" (http://www.un.org). This right has developed to include personal data exchange in business, government, and trade. Confidentiality of medical information goes beyond the patient-provider relationship. In the age of computers and information technology, confidentiality is harder to maintain. Health care information is available not only to the health care providers but also to any individual who has access to medical records, such as employees of health insurance companies. Yet a careful provider would not keep sensitive information on records that can be made available to others."

Health Insurance Portability and Accountability Act

In an attempt to protect the privacy of health information, the U.S. Congress passed the *Health Insurance Portability and Accountability Act (HIPAA)* of 1996 to aid in maintaining confidentiality of electronic records; however, this act also protects written and oral information. Canada has also taken steps to protect personal health information by recommending amendments to the *Criminal Code of Canada* for breaches of privacy (Health Canada, 2002). Confidentiality is an ethical concern in dental hygiene practice; it is also a legal concern.

PORTABILITY/TITLE I   The first part of HIPAA, Title I, guarantees that workers and their families are allowed to continue health insurance when they change or lose their jobs. This means that group health plans could not deny coverage or charge more for it because of past or present poor health. Also included are limiting the degree that preexisting conditions could be excluded from coverage, giving the right for small employers and those who lost job-related health benefits to buy heath insurance, and guaranteeing the renewal of insurance regardless of the health of anyone included in the policy (Ring, 2003, p. 22).

ACCOUNTABILITY/TITLE II   The second part of the act, Title II, became effective on April 14, 2003. In particular, HIPAA protects identifiable health information or *protected health information*, known as PHI, that could identify an individual. That is, PHI is information through which, if known, the identity of the patient can be recognized. This act outlines the handling of health information into three major sections: privacy standards, patients' rights, and administrative requirements. It should be noted that "if a state has a privacy law that is stronger than HIPAA's privacy rule, it will supersede HIPAA" (Ring, 2003, p. 23).

ELECTRONIC TRANSMISSION   *Privacy standards* ensure that the minimal necessary information is to be used and disclosed, thereby protecting a patient's identity and health information. Anyone or any organization, such as health plans, health care clearinghouses, and health care providers that transmit standard transactions in electronic formats are considered *covered entities* (Meyer & Schiff, 2004, p. 1). So a dental hygienist, dental office, or other entity providing health care is considered a "covered entity" and may use and disclose PHI for treatment, payment, and other activities. Other activities are sometimes referred to as "other operations" and include, for example, quality assessment. (The terms *treatment, payment,* and *health care operations* are identified at times by the acronym TPO.)

If one can "deidentify" protected health information, that is, make the information incapable of identifying a specific individual, one can disclose this information without consent or authorization. A patient must also be given written documentation (Notice of Privacy Protection) regarding how the information will be used and what rights he or she has in regard to one's own individual health information. This document must be signed by the patient and kept in the patient's file. According to PHI, a patient's information is to be disclosed only to the degree necessary—either to provide treatment or to arrange for payment (Ring, 2003, p. 26).

EXCEPTIONS   If PHI is used for other reasons, these reasons must be disclosed to the patient. The act ensures that patients' information is not given or sold to businesses. However, in cases of emergency, PHI can be released without the patient's permission. There are situations where the law requires confidential information to be given without the consent of the individual, such as in cases of abuse, communicable disease, fraud investigation, and gathering statistical data.

The HIPAA regulates the activities of a *business associate,* which is a person who performs a function or activity on behalf of a covered entity. Examples of business associates— or those who create, transmit, receive, or maintain PHI—are vendors, auditors, attorneys, consultants, billing services, transcriptionists, and practice management companies. Covered entities are required to obtain business associate contracts or written assurances that the business associate will safeguard electronic PHI (Meyer & Schiff, 2004, p. 44). Other employees, such as janitors, whose jobs do not require looking at health information, are not considered business associates.

PATIENTS' RIGHTS   In addition to the patient's signing a document that outlines the privacy practices of how protected information will be used, the patient should also be made aware of other rights mandated by HIPAA. These *patient rights* include the ability to access medical and dental records, to request amendment to medical and dental records, to request an accounting of disclosures, and to file a complaint internally (i.e., with the covered initiate) or with the Office of Civil Rights in the Department of Health and Human Services (Reynolds, 2004). A patient may also request restricting information that is shared within the organization or confidential communications such as phone calls or mailings. The act also outlines time-frame periods for responding to patients' requests and specifies protocols to be followed in that respect. The requests and responses must be in writing. Patients' rights according to HIPAA are outlined in Box 2-3.

FURTHER INFORMATION PROTECTION   Finally, to be in compliance with HIPAA, there is a set of *administrative requirements*.

- First, there must be a designated privacy officer and a designated contact person. In the dental office, this could be the same person or two different individuals, such as the office manager, dentist, dental hygienist, or dental assistant.
- Second, training should be provided to the employees. Recent graduates of dental hygiene or other health care professions have most likely received basic HIPAA training before entering internships or other clinical education. However, additional training may be required for specific protocols of the place of employment.
- Third, there must be safeguards in place to protect PHI.

BOX 2-3

Patients' HIPAA Rights

- Know how the information will be used
- Access medical and dental records
- Request amendment to medical and dental records
- Request accounting of disclosures
- File a complaint
- Restrict information that is shared
- Protocols for filing and responding to a complaint

Source: The Health Insurance Portability and Accountability Act of 1996

BOX 2-4

Updated Changes in HIPAA

- Business associates are governed by the same requirements as covered entities
- Individuals must be notified if there has been a breach of protected health information
- Patients can request copies of health record in electronic format
- Enforcement and penalties for HIPAA violations are increased

Source: The American Recovery and Reinvestment Act of 2009

STIMULUS PACKAGE   The American Recovery and Reinvestment Act of 2009, or stimulus bill, has made some changes in HIPAA by expanding privacy and security regulations. These updates to HIPAA are outlined in Box 2-4.

As confidentiality has always been important for the dental hygienists, many of the protocols are already in place. These include taking medical histories in a private area, not speaking about patients to family or friends, ensuring that other patients or personnel in nearby rooms or areas do not hear patients' conversations, shredding paper that contains patient information, and restricting the use of cellular phones (where others may accidentally overhear) when discussing patients. Other safeguards include passwords to open specific computer documents that contain PHI as well as methods to identify and track users and/or to detect activity of electronically transmitted information. Further information regarding compliance with HIPAA in dental/dental hygiene practice settings can be obtained from the American Dental Association's *HIPAA Privacy Kit.*

Societal Trust

Another core value that is incorporated into the ADHA Code of Ethics is **trust**. The code states, "We value client trust and understand that public trust in our profession is based on our actions and behavior" (American Dental Hygienists' Association, 1999, p. 17). The public, as individual patients and society in general, acknowledges dental hygienists' possession of specialized knowledge and skill. It is our ethical duty to ensure that this trust is maintained. However, this may be difficult when some members of society views health care providers as concerned with their self-interest more than with the patients' interests.

Society may form such a view when they suspect that providers act as "gatekeepers" for "for-profit" companies such as health care management organizations. In fact, many individuals believe that the present system has turned providers into employees eager to serve insurance companies and other employers more than they are interested in serving their patients. As a profession that values and relies on societal trust, dental hygiene must be alert to such misconceptions and must resist any attempt by for-profit organizations to endanger the interests of patients for financial gain. In the CDHA Code of Ethics, the concept of "trust" is incorporated in the principles of *accountability* and *professionalism* (Canadian Dental Hygienists Association, 2002).

DISCLOSING INFORMATION   Societal trust can also be jeopardized if the public perceives a breach of confidentiality. This is why dental hygienists and other providers should avoid providing any confidential information about their patients to a third party. If any practical need for revealing such information to a third party emerges, providers should weigh the benefit and cost of revealing.

Authorities investigating a crime may request access to records of some patients. In such situations, protecting the interests of society overrides the right to confidentiality. But there may be less obvious situations that are more difficult to judge. To deal with situations of this sort, the provider must examine two questions. First, is the harm of threatening societal trust in the profession outweighed by the benefit of revealing confidential information? Second, how can the amount of harm be kept to a minimum when it becomes ethically appropriate to break confidence (Purtilo, 1999, p. 156)?

Nonmaleficence

The core value **nonmaleficence** means to *do no harm* to others. Although the principle of doing no harm may not always seem sufficient for guiding human behavior, it is the most basic element in morality. In other words, it is a necessary condition for morality. If an action involves harming a person or a group, it cannot be considered moral. However, as already pointed out, there are situations that require providing tangible help for other people.

EXAMPLE   It is ethical not to interfere with the efforts of the Red Cross that are intended to relieve a famine in Africa. By not protesting or denouncing such efforts or by merely acknowledging them, one is demonstrating *nonmaleficence*. But suppose a person knows that the resources of the Red Cross and similar organizations are too limited to feed the hundreds of thousands who are dying of hunger. Would that person be acting morally by doing nothing other than approving of the goodwill of these organizations? In fact, a person who has a genuine interest in morality would feel compelled to participate in the effort of shipping or distributing food or donating money for famine relief. Sometimes by not doing anything, one may be doing harm.

Both beneficence and nonmaleficence are among the principles emphasized by the Hippocratic oath, although nonmaleficence is stressed as the most basic principle. The oath says, "*primum non nocere*," which means, "First, do no harm." More recent codes of ethics that are adopted by health care professions also deal with nonmaleficence as the foundation for medical ethics. The ADHA Code of Ethics states, "We accept our fundamental obligation to provide services in a manner that protects all clients and minimizes harm to them and others involved in their treatment" (American Dental Hygienists' Association, 1999, p. 17). Similarly, the IFDH Code of Ethics ensures that the dental hygienist uses "technology and scientific advances [are] compatible with the safety, dignity and rights of people" (IFDH, 2003, p. 3). In practice, dental hygienists act ethically when they apply all the measures that prevent harm, such as the standard precautions and thorough debridement. These two examples also demonstrate adherence to *standard of care*, which is closely related to nonmaleficence. Standard of care is discussed in Chapter 5.

Beneficence

The core value **beneficence** means doing what will *benefit* a person (e.g., a patient). Most ethical thinkers feel that doing no harm to other people (nonmaleficence) is not sufficient in all situations. A person who wants to do what is morally right will often find it necessary to offer active help to others. As dental hygienists, according to the ADHA Code of Ethics, we have "a primary role in promoting the well being of individuals and the public by engaging in health promotion/disease prevention activities" (American Dental Hygienists' Association, 1999, p. 17). This is consistent with the Report of the Surgeon General, which emphasizes that "oral health is essential to the general health and well-being of all Americans *and* can be achieved by all Americans" (U.S. Department of Health and Human Services, 2000b, p. 1).

Dental hygienists, as members of a profession that is meant to help the public, have obligations that extend beyond individual patients to society as a whole. In fact, societies have developed health care professions, including dental hygiene, to benefit their members. The principle of beneficence therefore underlies our profession and is also advocated by the CDHA Code of Ethics (Canadian Dental Hygienists Association, 2002). Furthermore, the IFDH Code of Ethics suggests: "The dental hygienist's own personal interest, if in conflict with her/his professional obligations should b e declared and resolved for the well-being of the client" (International Federation of Dental Hygienists, 2003, p. 2).

COMMUNITY BENEFICENCE   Dental hygienists are becoming more involved in public service and do not limit their efforts to providing care for private patients. They manage and operate programs in rural and remote areas and offer care to residents of nursing homes and geriatric facilities. Many hygienists also volunteer in preventive projects that are intended to help members of their communities, particularly of the less privileged. Fluoridation programs are examples for these projects. Such contributions to society show that the profession of dental hygiene is primarily guided by the principle of beneficence. Another form of beneficence is *pro bono*, which is donating one's services. A dental hygienist who donates time and skills to a public clinic or who arranges with the employer to treat those unable to pay is practicing the ethical principle of beneficence.

Justice

The core value **justice** can be defined as *fairness*. In the ADHA Code of Ethics, justice and fairness are considered together as one core value. The code states, "We value justice and support the fair and equitable distribution of health care resources. We believe all people should have access to high-quality, affordable oral health care" (American Dental Hygienists' Association, 1999, p. 17). This position is concerned with individuals and social groups. It emphasizes that patients should receive the same quality of care regardless of their socioeconomic status, ethnicity, education, or ability to pay. The concept of justice has been discussed in Chapter 1 and will be discussed further in Chapter 6.

Veracity

The core value **veracity** means telling the *truth*. According to the code, "We accept our obligation to tell the truth and assume that others will do the same. We value self-knowledge and seek truth and honesty in all relationships" (American Dental Hygienists' Association, 1999, p. 17). Truthfulness is a very important component in professional ethics. It is often in the best interest of the patient to know about his or her condition. Partial disclosure may lead to false hopes or unnecessary despair. Incomplete information, such as not telling patients of a less expensive option for treatment, may also generate financial or practical problems for patients. More important, withholding truth from patients can threaten the trust between the patient and provider. As discussed in Chapter 3, full disclosure of pertinent information is important for informed consent.

DECEPTION   Occasionally, a health care provider finds that withholding truth would serve the patient's interests more than truthfulness. In that case, it may be justified not to be truthful with the patient, at least temporarily. This kind of "therapeutic deception" is referred to as the *therapeutic privilege*. However, this practice should be limited to cases that definitely require it. Telling a patient that local anesthesia will eliminate any discomfort may be deception if the patient is not also told that pressure will be felt or that there may be discomfort as the anesthesia wears off. Both telling a child that dental treatment will not hurt when in fact it may and telling an adult that the only treatment option is the one covered by insurance when in fact there are other options are examples of deception. As stated in the IFDH Code of Ethics: "Truthfulness builds trust" (International Federation of Dental Hygienists, 2003).

ADDITIONAL ETHICAL PRINCIPLES

In addition to core values, other ethical principles may be found in professional codes. These, like core values, guide the dental hygienist in everyday treatment decisions and access-to-care issues. Awareness of the role ethical principles play in legislation, resource allocation, and other initiatives is essential for the dental hygienist. Application of these principles will aid the dental hygiene profession to continue working toward society's oral general health

Fidelity

The ethical principle **fidelity** is closely related to veracity, trust, and confidentiality. Fidelity means that the health care provider will be *faithful* to promises and obligations, will abide by rules and regulations, and will meet all reasonable expectations. In addition, fidelity means that the health care provider will act as a fiduciary, or a person who will act in the best interest of the patient. Although fidelity is not listed as a core value in the ADHA Code of Ethics, it is implied by other explicitly stated principles, such as trust and veracity.

Parentalism/Paternalism

The ethical principles **parentalism** and **paternalism** are used synonymously to denote acting like a parent with the intent to protect or enhance the interests of a person at a time when that person is unable or unwilling to protect his or her own interests. In such a situation, the autonomy of the protected person is restricted and his or her freedom of choice ignored or suppressed. The most acceptable form of paternalism is practicing natural parenthood, where parents do what is in the best interest of their children. Paternalism becomes a problem when the person on whose behalf another person is acting is a competent adult. Because competent adults can know what is useful or harmful for them, they need no other person to decide on their behalf. Indeed, a person who volunteers to make good decisions for competent adults would be violating that adult's autonomy.

Case Study Follow-up #2

What are some actions you, as the dental hygienist, could take to help the 15-year old patient in the case study?

PROVIDER AS PARENT   Does it follow that every act of paternalism is wrong? Suppose that a nurse saw a person in the clinic suffering from low blood pressure and circulatory collapse. He or she thinks that this patient needs urgent admission to the hospital to save his or her life, but the patient refuses. It is apparent that his or her refusal is the result of poor circulation, which causes impaired judgment and mental confusion. Should the nurse make a paternalistic decision and send the patient to the hospital without delay despite his or her protest? One is inclined to say yes, but it is difficult to justify forcing people to get treatment when they do not want to. However, knowing that acute illness frequently impairs the capacity to think soundly seems to be a good reason for an exceptional violation of autonomy. Furthermore, the nurse is not infringing on the patient's autonomy except to preserve the right to life. In normal circumstances, the patient would readily accept admission for treatment. So emergencies and temporary impairment of judgment may validate paternalistic actions on behalf of competent adults. Most well-intentioned paternalistic acts toward incompetent patients and patients who are considered minors are justifiable.

In dentistry, a patient may be told what a treatment will be but may not be given a choice. For example, a dentist may decide what type of material and procedure will be used for a restoration without telling the patient the other options for restorative treatment. By telling the patient only what the dentist feels the patient needs to know, and by withholding other information, the dentist has made a paternal decision and has violated the autonomy of the patient.

GOVERNMENT AS PARENT   In many situations, paternalism is practiced not by individuals but by institutions or governments. There are, for example, laws that prohibit the use of recreational drugs with the intent to protect people—even competent adults—from addiction and consequential hazards. In most states, the law requires all drivers and passengers to wear seat belts to protect them from injury in traffic accidents. Both examples reflect paternalistic settings where the state is acting on behalf of citizens to protect their interests. Yet some competent citizens do not want that protection and feel that they should be allowed to choose whether they use drugs or fasten seat belts. The state seems to such individuals an oppressive agency that restricts their freedom and denies their autonomy. However, the consequences of addiction and serious accidents are not limited to the individuals who choose to harm themselves.

EXAMPLES   Society shares the cost incurred by the unsound choices that some of its members make. It would be justified, at least for this reason, to accept particular forms of institutional (impersonal) paternalism. In fact, the most obvious form of institutional paternalism in the United States is the Food and Drug Administration. This agency decides for us which drugs are safe and which are risky. It limits our freedom of choice but at the same time protects us from potential harm. In public dental health programs, water fluoridation benefits the public and protects against caries. However, some citizens feel that this is forcing fluoride on individuals and think that it may even be detrimental to the health of the public. But the fluoridation program is still implemented to protect the teeth of most people. Mandatory vaccinations protect the general population. More recently a new paternalistic regulation has emerged: *Smokefree States*, where the government—not the owner or customer of a business—decides that there is no smoking inside a building or within a given amount of outdoor space in order to prevent diseases caused by secondhand smoke.

Utility

The ethical principle **utility**, or the *usefulness* of an action, underlies the theory of utilitarianism (see Chapter 1). The utility principle encompasses beneficence and nonmaleficence but goes beyond them. It is needed because neither beneficence nor nonmaleficence alone can solve the conflicts and competing needs in society.

EXAMPLE   A group of dental hygienists want to help the elderly poor in rural areas of their county to get sufficient preventive care. Guided by beneficence, the group considers sending three hygienists each week to a different remote area to take care of its elderly residents, but the funds they are able to raise will not cover all the expenses of the project. Some suggest transferring part of a fund that is intended for serving patients in urban nursing homes. Others disagree because the needs of urban nursing home residents are equal to those of rural residents. In such a situation, beneficence alone cannot tell the hygienists whether any group deserves more funds than the other. It can only tell them that it is morally good to help both groups. Similarly, nonmaleficence would not offer the needed answer. But the utility principle can be a reliable guide in that context. The utility principle would tell this group of dental hygienists to look for the action that benefits most nursing home residents.

RESOURCE ALLOCATION   The principle of utility is required to assess and rank the needs and wants of individuals or groups and to help determine social priorities. It can offer answers to questions about how to allocate resources and how to deal with the various needs of different sectors of society without causing significant harm to any sector. In effect, the principle imposes a social duty on us all to use our resources to do as much good as possible. That is, we must do the most good overall even when this means we are not able to meet all needs in a particular area (Munson, 1996, p. 36).

    When health care providers confront important decisions, they should consider the benefits and the burdens of each available choice. They should try to realize the greatest benefit and the least harm for their patients and community. The utility principle is useful not only for making choices and decisions regarding issues pertaining to groups but also for issues that concern individuals. For example, this principle can guide us to determine whether the risk of a diagnostic test outweighs the benefit of the information it provides.

PUBLIC HEALTH   Rights of individuals and the needs of the community are apparent in the field of public health. As dental hygienists expand their roles and the public health component becomes more vital through access-to-care and advocacy initiatives, they should explore the balance within the principles of beneficence, nonmaleficence, autonomy, and justice. Box 2-5 outlines the relationship of ethical principles to public health.

BOX 2-5

Public Health Ethical Principles

• Beneficence	Protection of individual welfare and promotion of the common welfare
• Nonmalficence	Weighing risks and potential harms of interveterventions against benefits for individuals and public
• Autonomy	Individual freedom in political life and personal development
• Justice	Distribution of resources, maximizing benefits to underserved, and equality of services

(Coughlin, 2009, p. 29)

Summary

Professional ethical behavior is guided by ethical principles and core values found in codes of ethics. The Code of Ethics of the ADHA identifies seven core values: autonomy, confidentiality, societal trust, nonmaleficence, beneficence, justice, and veracity. Similarly, the CDHA's Code of Ethics has similar principles of beneficence, autonomy, privacy and confidentiality, accountability, and professionalism. Other ethical principles include justified paternalism, utility, and fidelity. In some situations, these values conflict with each other, leading to ethical dilemmas. The right of patients to autonomy (i.e., to decide for themselves how they can be treated) should be respected by health care providers. However, in specific circumstances, this right may be restricted for the patient's benefit (e.g., with incompetent patients and in emergencies). The U.S. government legislates confidentiality through HIPAA.

Critical Thinking

1. Develop a code of ethics for dental hygiene students to follow while treating patients and interacting with fellow students and faculty.
2. Compare the newly developed student code of ethics with the ADHA or CDHA Code of Ethics.
3. Report on a situation that you encountered in the clinic where you were forced to make a decision between conflicting actions. Determine which core values or ethical principles were involved.
   a. What ethical principles or core values are similar? Which ones are different?
   b. If you were to develop a universal Code of Ethics for dental hygiene students, what elements would you include and why these specifically?
4. Refer to the case study at the beginning of the chapter, how can you (the dental hygienist) maintain the ethical principles of trust and fidelity with that patient?
5. As a health care provider, what are your responsibilities according to HIPAA standards?

CHAPTER 3

Informed Consent

OBJECTIVES

After reading the material in this chapter, you will be able to

- Discuss the criteria necessary for informed consent.
- Relate conditions for *not* obtaining informed consent.
- Compare the ethical principles found in codes of ethics, informed consent, patients' bill of rights, and other documents related to patient care.

KEY TERMS

Assent   Patients' bill of rights   Surrogate

Informed consent

INTRODUCTION

A patient's acceptance (or refusal) of a line of treatment based on the information provided by a health care provider is **informed consent**. Patients are becoming more aware of treatment options as partners in their health care decisions. This chapter will discuss the evolution of informed consent and the factors that need to be considered for patients to have self-determination about the health care they receive.

Case Study

You are informing your patient about the details of a crown procedure. She asks you about the possibility of recurrent decay, pain, or any other complications resulting from the crown as opposed to having the tooth extracted or a large amalgam restoration. Worried abut her refusing this recommended treatment option, you tell her that she should not worry because the dentist is an expert in this procedure.

As you read this chapter, consider the following: What information is missing for the patient to consent to the crown procedure? What ethical principles are involved with the information you are presenting to this patient?

HISTORICAL BACKGROUND

Simply, there are two sides to informed consent: being *informed* and giving *consent*. The patient is provided sufficient information about his or her condition and the available treatment options. Then the patient is allowed to discuss these options with the provider and to choose the most suitable treatment alternative. Informed consent allows the patient to make informed choices regarding treatment or care, and also includes the patient's right to refuse treatment.

The notion of informed consent was narrow and restricted until a few decades ago, when some court decisions triggered interest in reexamining and widening this notion. In the past, informed consent consisted of a patient signing, before surgery, a form stating the name of the operation and the risks associated with it. The purpose of these forms was twofold:

- Telling the patient about the nature of the procedure and its advantages and risks
- Ensuring legal protection for the practitioner if one of the mentioned risks occurs.

That context covered informed consent requirements at that time. The practitioner was acting ethically by doing what was *right* for the patient (i.e., what he or she considered to be in the best interest of the patient).

The concept of informed consent is not merely obtaining documented consent from a patient. Rather, it is considered a well-intended discussion between a provider and a patient, informing the patient about every relevant aspect in the proposed procedure, the alternative procedures, and the points that the patient should consider while opting for a particular procedure. The provider is no longer a paternalistic authority who decides what is best for the patient.

Giving Information

At first thought, the concept of informed consent may seem easy to understand: a practitioner tells the patient what will be performed and the patient agrees. But other aspects need to be considered. The following are only a few examples of countless questions surrounding informed consent. In fact, the concept of informed consent is multidimensional and involves substantial legal (e.g., negligence) and moral (e.g., patient's autonomy) issues.

- To what extent should the patient be informed?
- Should the explanations offered to patients involve technical details?
- Should the uncommon adverse effects of a therapeutic modality be specified?
- Would a practitioner be legally protected if he or she warns patients that the probability of the elected procedure causing severe bleeding is only 1 in 300 and then a patient happens to bleed excessively from that procedure?
- Could the failure of obtaining an informed consent automatically free the practitioner of legal liability if the patient's health deteriorates because of his or her decision to withhold treatment?

BOX 3-1

Some Negative Expectations of Treatment

- **Unanticipated outcomes** may have nothing to do with error, standard of care, or malpractice and may in some cases be positive outcomes rather than negative outcomes (Healthcare Providers Service Organization, 2004, p. 4).
- **Material risk** is "a risk that a 'reasonable person' would consider in determining whether to proceed with the proposed treatment" (Darby & Walsh, 2010, p. 1197).

Giving Consent

It may appear that by the mere action of entering your operatory, a patient is demonstrating informed consent, for if the patient had at least second thoughts about receiving your treatment, he or she would not be there. Yet this patient is likely to be demonstrating trust in a provider rather than consent. Meanwhile, not every act of consent is an informed consent. Patients should clearly know exactly what they are consenting to and what they can expect from the offered choice of treatment. They also need to be told about possible hazards and adverse effects. These include unanticipated outcomes and material risks as described in Box 3-1.

Patients' actions that demonstrate trust in their providers must not be interpreted as consent. Likewise, signing the Notice of Privacy Protection as mandated by the Health Insurance Portability and Accountability Act of 1996 (HIPAA) is not to be interpreted as informed consent for treatment (see Chapter 2). The importance of a clear and concise explanation of the treatment plan so that both the dental hygienist and the patient know what is expected at each appointment cannot be overemphasized.

Rights and Duties Involved in Informed Consent

So far, it has been implied that patients have a right to be informed and to make an independent decision whether to accept or reject a procedure or treatment strategy (recall the discussion of rights in Chapter 1). We have seen that people have basic rights, which include the right to life, autonomy, and fair treatment. Where the right to informed consent would be placed? This right is derived from the right to autonomy. If patients are granted freedom of thought and action, they should be enabled to choose the alternative treatment modality that they find appropriate for the circumstance. But to do that, this patient should be educated to carefully evaluate the available modalities and select the most suitable one. As already discussed, every right has a corresponding duty. And the patient's right to informed consent entails the duty of health care providers to adequately inform and advise the patient and not to try to influence any decision for reasons other than the patient's best interest. This is how the issue of informed consent relates to ethics.

Case Study Follow-up #1

- Did the patient have her questions answered?
- Was the dental hygienist influencing the patient's decision?
- Were options given other than the crown?
- Is the patient being told the advantages and disadvantages of an extraction, a crown, or an amalgam restoration?
- Is the patient being asked to trust and not consent to treatment?
- What other factors should be considered for *informed consent*?

EVOLUTION OF THE CONCEPT OF INFORMED CONSENT

The Hippocratic oath and code of ethics, which are intended for health professionals, emphasize the ethical principles of *beneficence* (doing what will benefit the patient) and *nonmaleficence* (doing no harm). Historically, practitioners made decisions on the basis of benefiting and not harming the patient. This practice, which is as old as the dawn of the art of healing, implied that physicians (or healers) act from benevolence toward their patients and that patients, in return, entrust them with their lives. Consent in that context was not really informed but rather was based on faith in the competence and dedication of the practitioner, that is, a belief that the practitioner knows best what should be done to treat each patient. In other words, informing patients was regarded as redundant and therefore not a right that patients were entitled to have. So the idea of informed consent is relatively new.

Types of Consent

There are three basic forms of consent: implied, expressed, and written. Patients opening their mouths for examinations without actually stating or signing forms that explicitly say that they agree to be examined are communicating an *implied consent* to the providers. Although they do not explicitly state their consent, they act as if they agree to be examined by the providers. The patient orally agreeing to a recommended procedure is *expressed consent*. An example of *written consent* would be the patient signing a statement authorizing the provider to perform a suggested procedure. For all these forms of consent to be ethical and legal, the patient must be informed about the procedure and must have the opportunity to comprehend and evaluate the risks and benefits of the suggested treatment (Wilkins, 2009, p. 376). Box 3-2 lists the three types of consent.

BOX 3-2

Forms of Consent

- **Implied Consent**—Non-verbal or unwritten agreement to a procedure
- **Expressed Consent**—Oral agreement to a procedure
- **Written Consent**—Signed agreement to a procedure

BOX 3-3

Assumptions of Harm-avoidance Model

- Patients do not want to know or to participate in making decisions about their treatment. (Perhaps it is true that some do not want to, but it would be wrong to generalize.)
- Patients would not understand the information anyway.
- The provider always knows what is in the best interest of the patient, making it unnecessary to get the patient involved and further complicate matters.
- The provider has both the authority and the appropriate medical knowledge to prescribe certain treatments to the patient, who has an obligation not to dispute their validity.
- Patients are, in most instances, extremely uninformed about their health, which makes it rather tedious, costly, and time consuming for providers to discuss treatment in any detail.

(Switankowsky, 1998, p. 37)

Harm-avoidance Model

In modern times, societies introduced measures to protect patients from unfounded trust in their health care providers. They introduced elaborate systems of licensing and assessing the competency of professionals. However, the "beneficence–nonmaleficence" practice continued to govern the relationship between patients and health care providers. This construal of consent as trust dependent was the basis of the *harm-avoidance model* of informed consent, which was introduced many decades ago. In this model, there is an obvious underestimation of the duty to inform the patient adequately as risks and benefits were left out. Thus, it has recently been modified. The reluctance of providers in the past, when the harm-avoidance model was still popular, to disclose information is possibly explained by *assumptions* that health professionals made (see Box 3-3). Therefore, in the harm-avoidance model, the practitioner adopts *paternalism* and the patient accepts that. As you may recall from our earlier discussion of the concept of autonomy and paternalism do not go together. Indeed, paternalism infringes on autonomy.

Examples

Another drawback inherent in the harm-avoidance model is that it encourages—or at least justifies—deceiving patients in order to motivate them or enhance their compliance. For example, a practitioner who hopes to benefit and protect a cancer patient may tell the patient that he or she has a chronic benign disease so that the patient does not abandon treatment out of despair or refuse a major surgery that could slow down his or her cancer. Similarly, a provider may give false information to his or her patient, either explicitly or by hinting about a prognosis of the severe disease, to protect the patient from depression and anxiety.

In the dental setting, a dentist may tell a patient with periodontal disease that a proposed surgical procedure will cure him or her totally to motivate the patient to accept the procedure. However, the dentist knows very well that this procedure will only improve the periodontal status, not cure the patient's the condition (as other factors are involved in periodontal disease that can not be controlled by surgery alone).

In the first example, the provider ignored, even denied, the *patient's right* to decide whether he or she wanted radical therapy or merely symptomatic relief. In the second example, the provider denied the patient's right to decide which practical arrangements he or she needs or wishes to make before dying (e.g., paying debt or modifying a will). In the third example, the provider denied the patients right to autonomy (i.e., to decide for himself or herself) acted from seemingly moral and legitimate principles. They were literally applying the beneficence and nonmaleficence principles. To accomplish their seemingly ethical goal (i.e., keeping their patients healthy for as long as possible), they ignored the patients' wishes and thought that it was justifiable to deceive them. But this paternalistic attitude toward informed consent, which permits the provider to determine which information to convey to patients or to withhold from them, is no longer accepted. As can be easily seen, paternalism ascribes unlimited authority to the provider and restricts the autonomy of the patient. There are exceptional situations, however, in which it is morally acceptable to hide information from certain patients.

Autonomy-enhancing Model

Autonomous individuals have control of their own lives and independently make their choices and decisions. This does not mean that providers are not supposed to advise their patients or recommend certain choices to them. It only entails that providers should not ignore the wishes and preferences of their patients and should avoid attempting to strongly influence patients' decisions after sufficiently educating them about the probable outcomes of each choice. As a result, the provider in the autonomy-enhancing model is not an authority but rather a *partner* in the process of deciding what is best for the patient. The provider in the autonomy-enhancing model does not have a passive role., but educates the patient on treatment options. Such a role limits paternalism and emphasizes participation and respect for patients' autonomy.

EXCEPTIONS TO THE RULE

A challenging question arises at this point. Can there be exceptions to the rule that informed consent must be obtained before treating a patient? What if the patient is not mentally competent and cannot make the best choice for himself or herself? What if the patient's condition was so critical that any time spent in obtaining informed consent would be at the expense of his or her life? The answer is that, like any known rule, the informed consent rule has a few important exceptions.

MENTALLY INCOMPETENT   If the patient is mentally or psychologically compromised or is experiencing a severe physical illness that diminishes his or her judgment, he or she cannot produce a truly informed consent. In that case, a legal representative, or **surrogate**, should be involved and should participate with the provider in decision making. This precaution prevents the undesirable scenario where a provider, who knows little about the social, financial, or family background of the patient, makes decisions that, despite the good intentions behind them, could disrupt the life of the patient. Other times, the caregiver is informed of treatment options and participates in the decision making. For example, a mentally incompetent patient with a dental abscess may refuse treatment for fear of more pain. The dental practitioner should involve his or her parent or guardian in the decision making.

EMERGENCY   Suppose that the patient was in critical condition and that talking with a surrogate will result in delaying urgently needed treatment. What could be done in such a case?

BOX 3-4

Exceptions to the Rule: Examples

There are situations, however, that are more complicated than the situations of mental incompetence and emergencies. Suppose that the patient is a competent adult woman who tells her provider that, no matter what, she will never accept a treatment that causes her to lose her hair. Unfortunately, the most effective treatment for her severe and life-threatening condition is a chemotherapeutic compound that leads in most cases to hair loss. Could the provider, with the intention of helping her recover from a serious disease, lie to her by denying that such a complication is feasible?

Consider a similar example. A clinician examines a male patient who fears having a hereditary fatal disease because his father and two brothers died of the same condition after years of suffering from both the illness and the side effects of treatment. This patient makes it clear to his provider that if he were found to have that disease, he would refuse any medication and die in peace. But the provider realizes that although the patient has the disease that killed his family members, it is still in its early stages and is likely to be mild and more responsive to therapy. If the clinician tells the patient the full truth, he would not accept any treatment, given his present state of mind. Could the clinician deceive this patient by telling him that his condition is superficially similar to but fundamentally different from his father's and brothers' disease?

Obviously, the provider should act from paternalism here. He or she must do what is best for the patient and what causes the least harm. The provider would be violating the patient's right to autonomy, yet he or she would be acting in good faith to enhance the patient's right to life. Adopting paternalism in this condition is morally warranted. Box 3-4 offers other examples for exceptions to informed consent.

For example, after being involved in a traffic accident, the patient suffers a fracture of the mandible but wants to postpone dental treatment. He or she wants to wait until the other, less serious injury to his shoulder improves. In that situation, the oral care provider (i.e., oral surgeon) can explain to this patient the importance of immediate oral surgery and can offer analgesic for the time being for shoulder pain. If the patient continues to resist, talking to the closest relative (i.e., spouse, parent, etc.) would be essential.

PATERNALISM   The questions posed in Box 3-4 are not easy to answer. In those and similar cases, the judgment of the provider should be individualized and adapted to the surrounding circumstances. If the woman who fears hair loss more than dying of a malignant disease seems an unreasonable person to the provider, the provider could stress the point that hair loss is a statistical finding, that she may be among the lucky people who escape this adverse reaction, and hair does grow back. If that attempt fails, the provider could refer the patient to a counselor.

The assumption here is that she is likely to change her attitude in light of professional counseling before the drug causes hair loss. A counselor may enable her to think more rationally about her life and health. Yet if counseling fails and she refuses to continue treatment, the provider has to withhold the drug and offer an alternative even if it is a less effective drug. But if she seems reasonable to the provider in her first visit, he could try a long session of education about the pros and cons of treatment versus preserving hair and then get an informed consent. There is no simple answer for such a situation, and the possibility of adopting a paternalistic attitude remains a viable, last resort.

TREATMENT REFUSAL   The case of the male patient who refuses treatment for a disease that killed his brothers and father can be handled on similar lines. Counseling, whether by the provider or a psychologist, could help. Any information withheld to avoid the consequences of psychological trauma should be fully disclosed on the patient's recovery from the initial psychological trauma. Otherwise, providers should not enforce treatment on competent patients who are not in life-threatening situations. At the same time, refusal to give informed consent should not be considered the end of discussion unless the patient was educated in depth about his or her condition. In other words, refusal of consent must be an informed refusal, and this is the provider's responsibility. Patients can refuse treatment, but they are entitled to know what would happen to them if they reject treatment and what they could gain if they accept treatment.

WAIVING INFORMATION   There are patients who prefer not to be informed. They find it upsetting to know about their condition in detail and think that they could deal better with it if they let the clinician make all the decisions. In other words, they opt for the harm-avoidance/paternalism context. Should these patients be forced to know about their condition and the recommended treatment? Individuals have the right to determine specific actions (as well as lifestyle choices) as they relate their health. This is entailed simply by the right to autonomy. Yet people are entitled to *waive* their rights. You may have the legal right to inherit your parents' wealth, but you choose to waive it so that your younger, disabled sister can get it and use it for her basic needs. The court cannot reject your waiver as long as it was made voluntarily. The same principle applies to waiving the right to be informed. In that case, the provider should accept the waiver and begin treatment.

AUTONOMY REVISITED   Another difficult question needs to be addressed. Suppose that you are treating a child whose parents do not believe in pharmacological therapy because their religion recommends prayer as the only valid method of healing. Would you let the young daughter suffer major problems because her parents refuse to consent to administration of needed drugs? Remember that the right to autonomy is purely individual. That is, each person has the right to determine his or her life but not anyone else's life. Remember also that parents are merely entitled to make decisions that enhance child's well-being. A parent, for example, cannot choose to let a child die when it is possible to save the life. This parent is entitled to commit suicide, but the parent is not entitled to kill a child because autonomy does not extend to children or other persons. Therefore, a provider facing such a problem should act in the best interest of the child and should seek legal help to stop the parents from harming their child. In such situations, the provider would be acting from benevolence (beneficence and nonmaleficence).

In dentistry, there are situations where parents neglect to give care to their children because they believe primary teeth are not important and that these teeth will be replaced. Providers of oral health care, in most cases, need to educate the parents about the role of primary teeth. Failing to seek the necessary treatment for their children, despite education by the dental hygienist and availability of the services (or absence of barriers), is neglect on the part of parents. In fact, neglect could be reported to social services as a form of child abuse (see Chapter 6).

BOX 3-5

Criteria for Informed Consent

- Competency of patient confirmed
- Understandable language used
- Diagnosis documented
- Need for treatment clarified
- Prognosis explained
- Alternative treatments stated
- Advantages/benefits clarified
- Disadvantages, risks, and side effects explained
- Cost specified
- Length of treatment discussed
- Provider of treatment specified

THE IDEAL CONTEXT

Full disclosure to the patient about his or her condition and providing helpful explanations of available treatment choices are essential for obtaining informed consent. Box 3-5 lists criteria necessary for informed consent.

Avoiding paternalism and allowing the patient to make reasonable choices is crucial. There are other precautions that can significantly help attaining the goal of effectively informing patients so that they can submit well-founded consent. One way to know if patients understand the treatment information is to ask them to describe to what they consenting. Box 3-6 outlines the information that must be given to the patient, the surrogate, or the parent/legal guardian in plain, understandable language.

BOX 3-6

Information for Informed Consent

- The diagnosis, or description of the problem.
- The nature and predicted course of the condition, both with and without treatment. The prognosis of untreated conditions and the possible cost of nontreatment, if known, should also be explained.
- Whether there is a need for certain procedures.
- The advantages, disadvantages, potential risks, cost, and long-term effects of all treatment alternatives as well as the estimated time for treatment and the expected effect on the patient's job performance during treatment.

These considerations are relevant to the daily practice of dentistry and dental hygiene. For example, in deciding to use an aesthetic material or an amalgam, the patient would have to know the advantage and disadvantage of each, such as the effect on the color of teeth or general appearance. A patient who smokes heavily and needs aesthetic restorations replaced several times because of staining may make a decision that differs from a nonsmoker's decision. This would also depend on the restorative material (i.e., less pourous composite material). Full disclosure will help both to decide. Similarly, patients may opt for a treatment that an insurance policy covers although such a treatment may seem less effective to the dental hygienist.

DELEGATION OF PROCEDURES   DeVore (1997) suggests that informed consent should also to include informing the patient about who will be performing the procedure (p. 60). In dentistry, there is a cross utilization of personnel for procedures. Unfortunately, patients are sometimes left unaware of the educational background, licensure status, and other qualifications of the provider who is performing a procedure. It is common that the dental hygienist, preceptor dental hygienist, certified dental assistant, and office-trained personnel may perform some of the same procedures. They have different education and may at times be performing procedures contrary to the Dental/Dental Hygiene Practice Acts. For example, compare your education as a dental hygienist to the education of a dental assistant: with four hours of education, the dental assistant in some states can legally apply pit and fissure sealants; with six hours of education, he or she can polish teeth; and with no educational requirement, the dental assistant can give fluoride treatments.

Most patients rely on dentists' judgment and trust that dentists will not delegate procedures to employees who are not capable of performing them or are legally not allowed to perform them. But this constitutes consent based on trust, not an informed consent. Consequently, patients in dental settings should be informed about the qualifications of personnel regarding a specific procedure and should be allowed to choose who is to treat them. Informed consent should also mean consenting to who will be providing the treatment, although this is not always the case. In this context, it would be appropriate to remind dental hygienists that they can facilitate informed consent while enhancing the profession of dental hygiene by informing patients about the educational standards of the dental hygiene profession.

Case Study Follow-up #2

Outline an *informed consent* discussion that you would have with the patient in this chapter's case study regarding a crown procedure. Compare it to the criteria outlined in Box 3-5.

DISCLOSURE IN THE OFFICE: PRACTICAL HINTS

In an effort to give the patient all the facts that are important in making a decision to accept or refuse a recommended treatment, the following are some other considerations that go beyond the benefits and risks. Remember what may not seem important to you as the provider could be the most important factor to the patient.

ESTIMATED TIME   In practice, the estimated time needed for completing treatment should be disclosed. Patients need to know how long a treatment would take, the number of visits, and the length of each visit. This helps the patient in scheduling appointments, dealing with insurance requirements, and arranging a payment plan. For example, patients who need extensive debridement will schedule several appointments over a relatively extended time with the hygienist. It is the dental hygienist's responsibility to inform the patient what the debridement procedure entails in terms of time and cost, even if the dentist or other authorized personnel, such as an office manager, has already given the patient a general idea. Adjunct procedures, such as oral irrigation, that are considered part of the consented treatment and any anticipated problems or discomfort after treatment should also be discussed with the patient before initiation of treatment by the dental hygienist. For treatment that is estimated to take over a year, the consent should be written.

ESTIMATED COST   Dental hygienists should be aware that cost is an important component of informed consent. Patients need to know the cost of treatment before they can commit to a lengthy treatment or confirm coverage with their insurers. Comparing costs of alternative treatments can help patients make a choice. For example, a patient may prefer an amalgam over an aesthetic restoration on the basis of cost. Similarly, cost may influence the decision of the patient to choose between having a crown or a large restoration.

For financial reasons, patients covered by insurance companies or health care management organizations need to know what procedures are covered by their plans. If dentists or dental hygienists recommend procedures or intervals that are not covered by insurance, patients should be helped to know the estimated out-of-pocket cost. For example, a health care plan may cover only one prophylaxis per year; however, the dental hygienist may recommend a more frequent debridement or prophylaxis schedule for a specific periodontal condition.

The patient should know the cost that is not covered by the health care plan before making a commitment. This situation is frequently encountered while practicing dental hygiene, and the prospective hygienist should be prepared to handle it. Likewise, if the dentist recommends an aesthetic restoration while the health care plan covers only amalgam, the patient should be aware of the difference in cost before agreeing to the recommended form of treatment.

TRUST   Communication is the core of informed consent. An open and trusting relationship needs to be developed between the patient and the health care provider. Trust cannot develop without full disclosure of all information. It is important for the hygienist to realize that disclosure may need to be repeated because many patients forget or pay insufficient attention at times. In addition, patients should be allowed enough time to adapt the cost to their financial situation. No patient should be made to feel that he or she must agree "right now." Patients should be given time to think over their decisions, as quick decisions may not be rational decisions (e.g., an atmosphere of unnecessary urgency may impair judgment).

VOCABULARY   Prospective hygienists have to recognize that some patients cannot understand technical or scientific language. Using medical terminology or giving a patient literature to read is not always appropriate. Frequently, published information is "user friendly" only for well-educated patients. The information required for obtaining consent has to be given in a way that is comprehended by the patient, and plain language is always preferable. Furthermore, for informed consent to be complete, the patient should be encouraged to ask questions, and the practitioner must ensure that the patient understands every aspect of his or her treatment plan. Occasionally, it may be appropriate to ask a patient to reiterate or repeat in his or her own words the conveyed information to verify complete understanding of recommended treatments. In summary, communication while obtaining informed consent should be based on mutual trust, which requires full disclosure, repetition, listening to the patient's preferences, and allowing time for decision making.

LANGUAGE   Many patients may not speak English nor have English as their first language. Likewise, patients may not speak the major language of the area in localities where English is a second language. For example, French may be the first language of people living in Quebec. In the United States, the Hispanic population is growing, and immigration is worldwide. Furthermore, oral health demands extend beyond the majority population. The dental hygienists must be cognizant of the fact that patients may not understand fully the information given to them in either oral or written form. Thus, a translator, appropriate literature, and cultural sensitivity are a must for informed consent to be valid.

REFUSING TREATMENT   Just as patients have a right to consent to treatment, they also have the right to refuse. Informed consent also means saying "no" to recommended treatment. For example, patients have the right to refuse treatment based on religious beliefs. Although these may not seem the decisions of "rational" individuals, health care providers must respect such decisions (Monagle & Thomasma, 2005, p.123). Christian Scientists, for instance, use individuals who are recognized as healers by prayer (as opposed to conventional medical treatment), and these individuals are recognized as practitioners and are reimbursed for their services through various insurance companies (DesAutels, Battin, & May, 1999, p. 11). Dental hygienists are expected to respect such beliefs and practices. However, when the patient refuses the recommended treatment, the hygienist must document this in writing (Pollack & Marinelli, 1988). If the hygienist thinks that rejecting conventional treatment may lead to deleterious effects on the patient's health, he or she should carefully inform the patient of such effects.

DOCUMENTATION   Documenting the refusal of the patient, information given to him or her (i.e., a recommendation or a list of consequences of refusal), and that he or she understood the risks of refusing care is equivalent to what is called an *informed refusal form*, which has legal importance. As with other documentation, the patient's refusal and the advice given to him or her should be dated and signed by the health care provider, the patient, and a witness. A copy of this completed form should be given to the patient, and another copy should be kept in the patient's file (Darby & Walsh, 2010, p. 378).

In addition, there should be documentation as to why the patient is refusing treatment (see Box 3-7). If the health care provider feels that he or she can no longer render any services to the

BOX 3-7
Treatment Refusal Documentation

Documenting the refusal of treatment should be noted in the patient's chart and should include:

- Provider's information given to the patient
- Patient's understanding the risks of refusing treatment
- Patient's reason(s) for refusing treatment
- Date and signature of patient, provider, and witness

If this refusal will mean ending the patient/provider relationship, then a letter should be sent to the patient.

patient based on the refusal to adhere to recommended treatment, then the patient needs to be informed of this in writing. Wilder (2004) uses the example of a patient refusing dental X-rays to illustrate the need for informing the patient about the reason for the recommended procedure, a letter to the patient informing him or her again about the recommended procedure and the need for it to provide "standard of care," and finally a dismissal letter sent by certified return receipt requested (p. 31).

INFORMED CONSENT AND RESEARCH

Most of the time, dental research is conducted in an institutional facility. As a dental hygienist who is employed outside of private practice, you may be involved in research with hospitals, public health departments, research centers, or other nontraditional dental hygiene practice locations. In addition, manufacturing companies may ask practicing dental hygienists to evaluate new materials on the market. Like all kinds of medical and health research, dental research may involve human subjects. This is required for advancing dental science and knowledge. But the rights of human subjects participating in research should be respected, including the right to full disclosure about the involved procedures. This is why informed consent is a necessary component of research.

RESEARCH PARTICIPATION   Research on human subjects has to be approved by an ethics or human subjects committee (or institutional review board) of the institution or agency that is sponsoring or conducting the research. Approving research on human subjects is conditional on ascertaining that the research project is needed and has scientific value and that it includes no risky procedures. Research should be considered the ethical principles of respect for persons and autonomy, beneficence and nonmaleficence, and justice (National Institutes of Health, 1979). In some cases, however, procedures involving a reasonable degree of risk may be allowed if it is believed that the potential benefit of such procedure outweighs its risk. A written consent form has to be signed by the participants (or parent, surrogate, or legal guardian). This form has to be dated and witnessed and should include all the components of informed consent for nonresearch procedures. For example, the nature of the study, procedures used, risks, benefits, and length of time should be specified. Participants are also given verbal information regarding the study. These same elements of informed consent should be provided in epidemiology and public health research (Coughlin, 2009).

Participants sign a consent form indicating that they have volunteered for the study and that they were not coerced into participating or prohibited from withdrawing from the study at any time. In addition, a contact person, such as the principal investigator, along with contact information, should be clearly indicated on the form. This ensures that a participant suffering from adverse effects of an experimental procedure can be promptly helped. Research should consider the ethical principles of respect for persons and autonomy, beneficence and nonmaleficence, and justice (National Institutes of Health, 1979).

ASSENT   Research involving children requires more than informed consent and permission from a parent or legal guardian. Depending on the research and the requirement of the specific internal review board or human subjects committee, both parents may need to give permission. The child must give **assent** or agreement to participate in research. An explanation of the research, procedures, and any discomfort or inconveniences must be given to the child in language he or she can understand. As with adults, participation must be voluntary and free of coercion, and children must have the opportunity to withdraw from the research at any time, even during the actual research procedure, and by just stating their desire to "stop" the procedure. State laws outline at what age or circumstances children are considered legally competent (e.g., age eighteen). For assent, the researcher should consider the age, cognitive development, and psychological state of the child. Assent from a child at age five would be quite different from assent by a child at age twelve or seventeen.

Some participants in research are paid for their time and effort. Details of payment as well as other material benefits should also be outlined. It is appropriate at this point to recall Kant's principle of treating persons as ends rather than as means (see Chapter 1). This principle should be followed when researchers decide to experiment on human beings.

USE OF PHOTOS AND OTHER RECORDING DEVICES

Informed consent is also necessary for voice, video, digital, or image recordings. These recordings are often gathered as part of a patient's file, research, teaching, presentations at professional conferences, publication in the professional literature (e.g., textbooks or journal articles), brochures, newsletters, telemedicine, and other uses. Patients must be given the opportunity to withdraw permission for the use of photo or recording and be assured that refusal to have the photo or recording will not affect medical care. Patients also must be told how the photo or recoding will be used, where it will be published, who to contact for questions, and where and for how long the photos or recordings will be kept. If the patient is a minor or incompetent, then permission must be obtained from the surrogate or parent or legal guardian. Asking for permission and informing the individual of the purpose(s) of the photo or recording takes into account the ethical principles of autonomy and confidentiality.

TAKING PICTURES   Photos may be published with a full view of the face. In an effort to conceal identity, the eyes can be blocked out or digital disguise used (Hood, Hope, & Dove, 1998). Individuals should be aware that when given permission for photos or other recordings to be used, it is possible that the images could be found later through e-mail, the Internet, and other computer transactions. Whenever possible, the photo that will be used should be shown to the patient, which is quite easy now with digital cameras and laptop computers. Often, models or actors may be used instead of the real patient in a scenario. Finally, photographs and recordings should take into consideration any misconceptions that could be interpreted through the photograph. It also should be culturally sensitive and should take into consideration the ethical principles of autonomy, nonmaleficence, beneficence, fidelity, and justice.

OBTAINING PERMISSION   In group events, it is best to talk with the person in charge of the event, state who you are and the purpose for taking pictures or recoding a video including those by cellular phones. If a picture is taken at a public event, it may not be necessary to obtain permission, as individuals would be expecting to have cameras and other media present. Photos or videotaping at a school setting may require input from the principal or other individuals, such as parents or legal guardians. As more opportunities are available for dental hygienists to work outside the private dental practice, they should become more knowledgeable about the use of photographs and other recordings that identify individuals. Box 3-8 gives an example for the use of photos.

BOX 3-8

Use of Photos Example

Consider, for example, the use of sealants with an elementary school-based sealant program.

- We may want to take photographs of the teeth to show the pre- and post-application of the sealant material.
- We may want to videotape the procedure to illustrate how the setup of the equipment in a school setting is different from or similar to that in traditional private dental practice.
- We may want to take photos to print a brochure that explains to parents the school-based sealant program. We may have media present to produce a public service news item on the local television station.
- We may take photographs for an article in a dental hygiene journal or for a poster presentation at a professional conference.
- We may have our community project with participants posted on Facebook or other Internet portals.

All these and many more situations require different levels of permission from various individuals.

DISCLOSURE BY INFECTED HEALTH CARE PROVIDERS

As discussed earlier, informed consent requires that patients be informed of all possible risks before agreeing to treatment. Does that also mean that health care providers infected with blood-borne viruses such as hepatitis B, hepatitis C, or HIV should inform their patients? It is possible that practitioners who do not adhere to strict precautionary measures infect their patients. In fact, the only documentation of a patient obtaining HIV from a health care practitioner has been in dentistry, although it was not possible to determine how the virus was transferred (Centers for Disease Control [CDC], 1991, 1998; Kessler, Bick, Pottage, & Benson, 1992, p. 666).

In the early 1990s, the CDC, the American Medical Association, and the American Dental Association issued recommendations for health care providers who were HIV infected. These interim recommendations stated that HIV-positive providers who perform invasive procedures should stop practicing or inform their patients of their status. These guidelines relied on the principle of nonmaleficence to protect patients from a provider who could potentially harm them.

GUIDELINES   The CDC's 1991 and 2003 proposed guidelines include adherence to universal (now termed *standard*) precautions and identification of *exposure-prone* invasive procedures, which are to be handled with utmost caution. It was decided that providers should know their HIV and hepatitis B status (although they are not required to disclose it) and abstain from performing exposure-prone invasive procedures on patients without discussing the matter with review panels (Centers for Disease Control, 1991, 2003; Glantz, Mariner, & Annas, 1992, p. 48). Thus, the responsibility for protecting patients was assigned to members of health care professions, and mandatory testing for health care workers was considered unnecessary.

Obviously, if these precautions are strictly followed, the probability of patients being infected by HIV- or hepatitis B–positive practitioners who know that they are seropositive would

BOX 3-9

CDC Recommendations for Infected Health Care Workers

- Use of standard precautions (*term universal precautions* is no longer used since 2003)
- No restriction for invasive, no exposure-prone, procedures provided that standard precautions and sterilization/disinfecting procedures are followed
- Exposure-prone procedures should be identified by organizations and institutions
- Knowledge of one's own HIV antibody and HBsAg status for performing exposure-prone procedures
- Infected health care workers should seek counsel from expert review panel regarding circumstances to perform exposure-prone procedures and notifying prospective patients
- Mandatory testing is not recommended

Source: Morbidity and Mortality Weekly Report 40 (RR08), 1–9 (publication date: July 12, 1991), and (RR17), 1–61 (publication date: December 19, 2003).

be very low. However, a provider who is unaware of his or her seropositivity status may accidentally infect a patient while performing an invasive procedure. It is likely that the guidelines will be further modified if more cases of transmission from clinicians to patients are discovered. Although these CDC recommendations do not specify (or list) hepatitis C, it is expected that those health care providers infected with hepatitis C should follow these same recommendations (see Box 3-9). Others recommend standard precautions be used and without restrictions on professional activity unless "epidemiologically linked to transmission of disease" (Darby & Walsh, 2010, pp. 86–67).

Canadian health care workers infected (or have history of positivity) with hepatitis B, hepatitis C, or HIV are expected to notify the provincial expert review panel through their regulatory or licensing bodies. This is considered an ethical responsibility of the infected health care provider. Those providers with hepatitis B may have their practice restricted (i.e., ability to do surgery modified). Health care workers infected by hepatitis C or HIV may continue to perform high-risk procedures. As in the United States, testing of all health care providers is not recommended, and confidentiality is to be respected (Public Health Agency of Canada, 1998).

The ethical question here is, which right takes precedence: the patient's right to safety or the provider's right to privacy? Proponents of patients' rights point to the right to safety of the patient and insist that it is the provider's duty to disclose his or her HIV status. Advocates of privacy argue that the likelihood of infection is so low that disclosure is unnecessary. Perhaps the recommendations strike a balance between both points of view, and time will show how adequate these recommendations are.

It is very important to realize that dental and dental hygiene procedures are exposure prone since they are invasive because of the use of needles for injections (local anesthesia) and sharp instruments (debridement, scaling, and root-planing procedures). Therefore, it is imperative that *clinical* dental hygienists be constantly aware of their own serologic status. A hygienist who turns positive is required to accept the judgment of a review panel and to disclose his or her status to patients. This is not only a legal issue but also—and primarily—an ethical one.

PATIENTS' BILL OF RIGHTS

Patients are guaranteed information regarding their care through informed consent. But also but through the **patients' bill of rights** informs them about the general principles of their care. This bill typically outlines what the patient can expect as a partner in his or her own health care. The wording of the bill may vary from one facility to another, but the fundamental rights are usually stated everywhere. The bill includes the patient's right to be informed and to accept or refuse treatment or participation in research. In addition, the bill assures patients that they are entitled to know who is treating them, which external agencies are affiliated with the facility providing care, and the rules regulating charges and payments. The bill also endorses the patient's right to know of any alternatives to the proposed treatment. Box 3-10 gives an example of patients' rights in terms of oral health care.

MEDICAL FACILITIES AND PATIENTS' RIGHTS   Private dental offices may or may not have their own patients' bill of rights (see Box 3-10). The patients' bill of rights is usually displayed in visible places, such as the reception area of a health care facility, but copies may also be distributed with other forms that the patient has access to, such as informed consent or "new patient introductory forms" (Dietz, 2000, p. 117). However, many clinics, hospitals, and other dental treatment centers display this bill as a part of their policy. For example, a dental clinic in a hospital may display the patients' bill of rights created by the American Hospital Association. Other organizations, such as the Canadian Dental Hygienists Association, have also developed documents outlining patients' rights (www.cdha.ca).

BOX 3-10

A Concise Version of Patients' Bill of Rights for Dental Hygiene Practice

We strive to consider *patients as partners* in their oral health care and in meeting their oral health care needs. As patients in our care, you can expect the following:

- You will be treated with respect, dignity, and courtesy.
- Information about your health will be confidential, and privacy will be maintained.
- You will be informed of length of appointments and fees before scheduling services. Appointments will be kept, and a reasonable fee will be charged. You will be made aware of insurance and payment arrangements.
- You will be kept informed of your dental and dental hygiene needs, progress of treatment, and any change in treatment conditions.
- You will be encouraged to seek alternative treatment, referrals, and second opinions when necessary.
- You will have access to your dental and dental hygiene records.
- You will have the right to refuse treatment.

Note: Adapted from Dietz (2000, p. 118).

PATIENTS' BILL OF RIGHTS ACT   Congress proposed the Patients' Bill of Rights Act of 1999 to help patients, as consumers, make decisions regarding health services and benefits. This legislation's intent was to help consumers obtain health coverage and increase the country's health care systems, quality of health, and research. (Patients' Bill of Rights Act, 1999). This act seeks to protect patients, as consumers, by expanding disclosure requirements, grievances, appeals, reviews, and genetic nondiscrimination provisions found in health care plans. Ideally, the act will promote better access to care and quality of care as patients are allowed to question treatment decisions, such as emergency room visits and referrals to specialists, determined by their health care plans and primary care providers.

Summary

Informed consent consists of two components: information for the patient and consent by the patient. The patient must be informed of the recommended treatment, its risks, and alternative treatments. Exceptions to informed consent occur in situations of emergencies and mental incompetence. Patients are also entitled to refuse treatment after being informed about its importance and about the consequences of refusal. Surrogate decision makers (i.e., parents or legal guardians) must be informed when patients cannot make decisions for themselves (e.g., patients in coma or children) and are supposed to consider the best interest of the patients. Patients may also waiver the right to informed consent; that is, they may not want to be involved in decisions regarding treatment. Applying the therapeutic principle, health care providers can also withhold information from patients if it is in the interest of the patients not to be told. There is controversy regarding the right of patients to know whether their health care providers are infected with HIV or similar infectious illnesses, but reasonable guidelines have been issued by the CDC and other agencies to protect patients without violating the privacy of providers. The patients' bill of rights provides additional assurances for patients about their entitlement to know about and accept or reject a recommended treatment. Individuals should also give informed consent for use of photographs and other recording information for research, publications, education, and other purposes.

Critical Thinking

1. List the criteria necessary to obtain informed consent from competent adults. How does this differ in situations involving (a) a minor (child), (b) an incompetent patient, (c) an emergency, and (d) a patient not giving permission for treatment?
2. Divide into pairs. Role-play the following activities:
   a. Ask for *informed consent* from a patient for dental hygiene periodontal therapy. This patient has never had debridement or prophylaxis treatment and has had limited restorative treatment. The patient comes from a background where one visited the dentist only if there was pain. There is heavy calculus and generalized pockets of 4 to 6 mm.
   b. Ask for *informed consent* from a parent for a minor to receive X-rays, pit and fissure sealants, and fluoride treatment in addition to the scheduled examination and prophylaxis.
   c. Ask for *informed consent* from a female patient of childbearing age for local anesthesia.
   d. Ask for *informed consent* from a fifty-five-year-old male patient for nitrous oxide–oxygen sedation.

3. Read the *patients' bill of rights* posted in your dental hygiene program. Are there any items that you would like to add?

4. Give examples or develop scenarios where it would be appropriate for the dental hygienist to apply the principle of paternalism through nondisclosure.

5. Compare a code of ethics with a patients' bill of rights. What ethical principles or core values are found in both?

6. You want to show your parents the involvement your dental hygiene program has in the community. You use your cell phone to tape the actions of your classmates in the recent *Give Kids A Smile Day*. What are your responsibilities before your post this video on the Internet?

7. Using the information in this chapter's case study, how should you address the concern the patient has with accepting the crown procedure?

CHAPTER 4

Decision Making

OBJECTIVES

After reading the material in this chapter, you will be able to

- Define the term *ethical dilemma*.
- List the steps involved in ethical decision making.
- Solve ethical dilemmas using a decision-making process.
- Determine core values and principles used to solve an ethical dilemma.
- Discuss the role of laws in determining alternatives for solving an ethical dilemma.

KEY TERMS

Decision making   Dilemma   Ethical dilemma

INTRODUCTION

Throughout our lives, we are faced with the necessity of **decision making**. Decision making is a process using critical-thinking skills to arrive at a judgment or conclusion. Before you entered dental hygiene, you made the decision to continue your education. Then you decided where to enroll. Later, as a student, you may have had to make the decision to work on weekends to support yourself. After graduation, you will make many other decisions. Life is full of situations that require decisions, and some decisions are difficult to make.

Dental hygienists make decisions daily. While treating patients, dental hygienists constantly are using critical-thinking skills. For example, they use decision making in selecting the type of fluoride to use for a patient with ceramic crowns. Although the majority of dental hygienists work under the supervision of dentists, dental hygienists are responsible for the dental hygiene treatment needs and dental hygiene care plans. As members of a profession, dental hygienists have autonomy in these decisions and should provide treatment that meets the acceptable *standard of care* for all dental hygiene procedures

At times, however, the decisions may not be easy. For example, the dentist's line of treatment and referral (or lack of referral) may conflict with the treatment plan designed by the dental hygienist. In this situation, the dental hygienist may choose to follow the suggestions of the dentist or ignore them and risk losing his or her job. Throughout this chapter, a case study will be used to demonstrate the decision-making process.

Case Study

The Medicaid-only clinic has a new "no-show" policy of three missed appointments without calling to cancel, and the patient will be released from the practice. The staff has been told that this rule is for everyone—no exceptions. The reasoning behind this new change is to limit the "down time" of the dentists. The clinic is solely operated by Medicaid reimbursements, and the dentists get paid whether or not they have patients scheduled.

There is a single mother with three children who have been missing appointments regularly. They are usually scheduled together and have broken eight appointments over the past six months that they have been patients at this clinic. The children have large treatment care plans that desperately need to be completed. The mother works many hours each week at a convenience mart and is commonly called in to work when someone else does not show up. She is the sole provider for her family, but she has parents who help watch the children when she is at work. They all live in a town 45 miles from the clinic, hence the reason for scheduling them at the same time. She does not have anyone, other than herself, who can take the children to their appointments.

She recently called the clinic manager, a registered dental hygienist/social worker, and was pleading her case to not release her children as patients from the clinic. She said that all of the other Medicaid clinics in the area have already told her they can no longer see the family owing to all of their missed appointments. The clinic manager explained the reasons for the new rule, and the fact that the clinic can never get in touch with the mother by phone to confirm the appointments. The mother explained that she buys minutes for her cell phone and sometimes does not have the money to do so. She is not allowed to take calls at work. The manager would like to keep seeing the children because of all the dental work they need but cannot allow them to keep missing appointments due to the loss of productivity.

As you read this chapter, consider the following: Would you continue to make appoints to treat these children? What ethical principles would you consider in your decision? How would you make your decision?

ETHICAL DILEMMA

A **dilemma** is a situation necessitating a choice between two equal, especially undesirable alternatives. An **ethical dilemma** may be defined as a conflict between moral obligations that are difficult to reconcile (Honderich, 1995, p. 201). For example, if a person has to choose either to buy a new car and be in debt for several years or to keep an old car and spend a lot of money on mechanical repairs, he or she is confronting a dilemma. Ethical dilemmas are challenges that require moral reasoning. Moral reasoning, in turn, needs to be guided by ethical principles. In this example, the single mother could use the utilitarian and beneficence principles to choose the arrangement that does the least harm to each involved party.

EXAMPLE   A person facing an ethical dilemma is a single mother whose elderly and disabled parents need her care but who cannot care for them and her children without giving up her full-time job. At the same time, she cannot quit her job before her children finish their education and are able to support themselves. This person, obviously, is not in a position to fulfill the obligations imposed on her in an adequate way. The dilemma she is facing is not practical but ethical because it involves the well-being of other persons and her duties toward them.

Dental hygienists may confront similar ethical dilemmas. There will always be situations that require satisfying multiple parties. The best interest of the patient is not always compatible with the interests of insurance companies, hospitals, dentists, or other care providers. The dental hygienist must take into consideration the conflicting interests of all parties. He or she may find that the amount of work needed for a nursing institution patient cannot be done without disrupting the budget of that institution. The scarcity of these funds leaves the dental hygienist in a dilemma.

Dental hygienists should be prepared to deal with ethical dilemmas in efficient ways. Like the single mother in the previous example, the dental hygienist needs ethical principles to resolve dilemmas. The core values or ethical principles (discussed in Chapter 2) found in the Codes of Ethics of the professional dental hygienists associations (American, Canadian, international, and one's own country) may be a good starting point in solving ethical dilemmas. They provide dental hygienists with general strategies of action that if followed are likely to lead to the most acceptable results. For example, they inform the dental hygienist of the importance of preserving societal trust in all situations.

When the best interest of the patient conflicts with the best interest of the public, the hygienist would have to find a compromise that furthers the patient's interests without jeopardizing public trust. For example, it may be in the best interest of some patients to use cosmetically appealing materials (such as ceramic inlays). But the public may not accept paying higher insurance premiums to cover the cost of such materials. In that case, the dental hygienist should balance the preferences of the patient with those of society. Otherwise, dental hygienists may lose the trust of the public.

However, the various codes of ethics do not provide guidelines for every situation. In fact, all codes of ethics are intended to reinforce and complement rather than to replace the reasoning capability of professionals. As a dental hygienist, you will need to use other means of problem solving when you face a dilemma. In addition to the code of ethics, you may draw on reasoning skills that you acquired throughout your life by socialization, previous experience, learning from role models, formal ethical education, and even *gut feeling* (or intuition). Dental hygienists facing ethical dilemmas use, in addition to the principles stressed by their code of ethics, advice from peers, legal advice, and their personal experiences. They also consider legal and administrative consequences while making decisions regarding ethical problems. However, the way an ethical dilemma is solved should in the end conform to the moral principles and core values discussed in previous chapters. Box 4-1 lists some factors used in decision making for an ethical dilemma.

Cobban et al. (2005) reported that the majority of senior dental hygiene students who witnessed unethical behavior in the clinical education environment felt uncomfortable challenging the individuals involved and discussing the situation (p. 71). Stern (2003), in her study of decision-making strategies, suggests that experienced clinicians consider the whole context as well as professional principles when resolving ethical dilemmas more than students do.

This shows that having practical and clinical experience improves the ability to deal with ethical questions.

BOX 4-1

Some Factors Used in Ethical Decision Making

- Professional code of ethics
- Advise from peers, lawyers, superiors, role models, etc.
- Intuition or gut feelings
- Personal experience and socialization
- Consequences of previously made decisions

Examples

EXAMPLE 1   Think about the following case scenario. A woman has been receiving *routine* care since childhood. She has now moved from her hometown and comes to your office as a new patient for her six-month dental hygiene prophylaxis. You initiate your appointment with a review of her medical history, radiographs, probing, and other assessment measures. This patient has generalized bleeding and localized pockets. You find heavy subgingival calculus, especially in the interproximal posterior regions. Your patient needs to return for another appointment. She questions why she needs to return and why you did a lot of "extras" before you started treatment with the ultrasonic scaler. She states that in the previous office, her appointments always were completed within one hour and that the dental hygienist always complimented her on how well she took care of her teeth.

This poses an ethical dilemma. Would you tell the patient that she had previously been given poor treatment that was not current with standard of care? Or do you continue to treat her in the manner she is accustomed to and compromise your treatment? The first choice may lead to a loss of societal trust in dental hygiene. The public expects dental hygienists to provide high-quality care. In addition, pointing to the faults of colleagues should be avoided whenever possible. At the same time, the second choice implies giving substandard care to the patient. Or, do you explain the reasons for these "extras" to a new patient as a means of obtaining baseline data? If you were the dental hygienist, how would you resolve this dilemma?

EXAMPLE 2   Consider a patient who is also a mother. She asks you to write an absentee form stating that she needs another appointment so that she can take a sick day from work to be with her child for a school recital. You know that it is morally wrong to lie, yet you appreciate how important it is to both mother and child that she attend the recital. Should you lie for the parent and arrange for the requested absence form? How would this lie be perceived? Should you suggest that the mother explain to her child how difficult it is to leave work and hope that the child will understand and accept the situation? What is your position on this situation? Would your position change if the mother will receive pay for a sick day but not for missing work for personal reasons?

EXAMPLE 3   The dental hygienist's care plan may conflict with the patient's insurance company's coverage plan, which may not cover the preferred treatment. In that case, the dental hygienist may decide to modify the plan to agree with the insurance policy or to let the patient decide whether to pay the extra cost. This former example, there was a conflict between two interpretations of the patient's best interest: one offered by the insurance company and the other by the dental hygienist. Is the conflict ethical or practical? The conflict arose between the administrative policy of the insurance company and the care plan. It was also a practical conflict because it concerned financial issues without endangering the patient's oral health. What is the role of informed consent in solving this dilemma?

EXAMPLE 4   Not all the conflicts that dental hygienists confront are technical or practical. They also meet with moral (ethical) conflicts. Suppose that the dental hygienist finds that his or her patient needs referral to a periodontist for an effective treatment but that the dentist does not like to refer patients whenever he or she could perform a useful but less effective treatment at the office. This hypothetical dentist may have reasons for withholding referrals. He or she may be interested in maximizing income or in practicing a technique that was recently learned. The dentist may be concerned that referred patients might lose their ties with the office and never come back. The situation here is not merely practical. It has a moral dimension. The basic issue is not the patient's best interest but rather the dentist's self-interest. The patient is treated not as an end in himself or herself but as means to generate income for the dental office or to benefit the dentist in another way.

EXAMPLE 5   Suppose that a patient has an old restoration that needs replacement but that the policy of the office is to prophylactically replace all old restorations regardless of their condition. The assumption here is that old restorations will eventually deteriorate no matter what. Should the dental hygienist volunteer to tell the patient that the benefit of replacing all old restorations at present is questionable and that the patient should make it clear to the dentist that he or she wants only defective restorations replaced? This hygienist faces two incompatible choices: to comply with the policy of the office or to give priority to the best interest of patients. This situation also has a moral aspect.

SOLVING ETHICAL PROBLEMS

It is important to realize that there are several factors that influence our decision making in solving ethical dilemmas. We do not acquire the ability to solve ethical problems and make ethically relevant decisions overnight. Rather, it is a gradual and lengthy process that begins even before reading about morality, taking a course in ethics, or studying the code of ethics appropriate for your profession. You may recall that you began to think about "good" and "bad" actions in your early childhood. You may also remember how parents and teachers tried to guide your reasoning about what is good or bad by examples and anecdotes or by simply giving you firm instructions.

The moral conscience has its roots in early life and is influenced by cultural elements. Modern social scientists have proposed theories to explain this process. Among these theories is Kohlberg's model of moral development, which gained remarkable popularity among students of ethics. It is useful to be acquainted with this model because it highlights the gradually evolving process that leads to acquiring the ability to make ethical decisions.

Kohlberg's Model

Lawrence Kohlberg (1967) suggested that there are three levels and six hierarchy stages to moral development (see Table 4-1). Each level has two stages, and each step must be reached before progressing to the next step. The three levels are preconventional, conventional, and

TABLE 4-1   Levels and Stages in Moral Development

Level I	***Preconventional Level:*** Moral values reside in external quasi-physical happenings, in bad acts, or in quasi-physical needs rather than in persons and standards. **Stage 1:** Orientation to punishment, obedience, and physical and material power. Rules are obeyed to avoid punishment. **Stage 2:** Naive instrumental hedonistic orientation. The child conforms to rules to obtain rewards.
Level II	***Conventional Level:*** Moral values reside in performing good or right roles and in maintaining the conventional order and the expectations of others. **Stage 3:** "Good boy" orientation designed to win approval and maintain expectations of one's immediate group. The child conforms to avoid disapproval. One earns approval by being "nice." **Stage 4:** Orientation to authority, law, and duty to maintain a fixed order, whether social, legal, or religious. Right behavior consists of doing one's duty and abiding by the social order.
Level III	***Postconventional, Autonomous, or Principled Level:*** Moral values reside in conformity by the self to shared or shareable standards, rights, and duties. **Stage 5:** Social contract orientation, in which duties are defined in terms of contract and the respect of others' rights. Emphasis is on equality and mutual obligations within a democratic order. There is an awareness of relativism of personal values and the use of procedural rules in reaching consensus. **Stage 6:** The morality of individual principles of conscience that have logical comprehensiveness, universality, and consistency. These principles are not concrete (like the Ten Commandments) but general and abstract (like the Golden Rule or the categorical imperative).

Source: Adapted from Oldenquist (1978) and Rich and DeVitis (1985).

postconventional. The basic assumption of his theory is that as individuals pass through these stages, they progressively utilize thinking and problem solving more than they utilize fixed rules to solve ethical dilemmas. But to reach the stage of thinking rather than just following fixed rules, one needs to gain cognitive development. Cognitive development means developing knowledge of the moral values and standards of one's group or society. Having such knowledge is essential for developing the ability to make moral judgments.

Kohlberg based this theory on his study of males of different ages, different socioeconomic backgrounds, and different cultures. His findings suggest that children tend to solve problems at a simple level, which he described as stages 1 and 2. Most adults, however, tend to operate at a more complex level, described as stages 3 and 4. But only 20% of the population was able to reach a higher level of moral reasoning, and not all of them reach the final stage in that level, which Kohlberg described as stage 6. He found that less than 10% of the adult population operates at stage 6. As dental hygienists, we should aspire to reach the final stage or the most advanced level of moral reasoning in general. This will enable us to solve moral dilemmas in the most rational way. But, as Kohlberg's research shows, not many people reach this final stage. It is plausible to suggest that what is needed for reaching the most advanced stage is the study of ethics.

Rest's Model

Among social scientists who tried to refine Kohlberg's model is James Rest. He suggested that developing cognitive dimensions to moral reasoning requires attaining other abilities, such as moral sensitivity, moral motivation, and moral character (Rest, 1986). While Kohlberg stressed cultural and societal influences, Rest emphasized the importance of education and personal experience. He pointed out that age and education had an effect on moral thinking; the older and more educated individuals tended to behave more morally.

This observation applies to dental hygiene students. In an important study, dental hygiene students who had more formal education were found to have more advanced moral reasoning ability than those who had less formal education (Newell, Young, & Yamoor, 1985). Bebeau, Rest, and Yamoor (1985) reported similar results with dental students: Third-year dental students reasoned at a higher level than first-year dental students, and faculty reasoned at a higher level than students. These studies support the notion that dental hygienists can better serve their clients (and society in general) by attaining the highest possible level of education, which should include ethical education. Dental hygienists should participate in lifelong learning and professional continuing education to help ensure the best care for their patients.

The awareness of the basic principles of morality, which are discussed in the opening chapters of this book, is very important for making sound ethical decisions. It would be useful for dental hygienists to reflect on this account and adapt it to the dilemmas that they encounter in their practice. It is particularly useful to capture its emphasis on the significance of having the desire and motivation to act morally in all situations.

DECISION-MAKING PROCESS

Decision making, as already defined, is a process that uses critical thinking to make a judgment or to reach a conclusion. Critical thinking is reasoning in an objective, organized, and logical manner. In clinical dental hygiene practice, we often use critical thinking to formulate a dental hygiene care plan based on the treatment categories: assessment, dental hygiene diagnosis, planning, implementation, and evaluation (Mueller-Joseph & Peterson, 1995, p. 2; Wilkins, 2009, p. 357).

Decision making in ethical contexts requires critical thinking. Like practical problems, an ethical problem or dilemma cannot be solved in a subjective or arbitrary manner. Good reasoning is our best tool for solving problems, whether they are clinical, scientific, administrative, or ethical. This is why dealing with ethical problems proceeds on lines similar to those followed in solving clinical problems in dental hygiene practice. It is important to bear in mind that "health decision-making involves two components: a technical decision requiring the judicious application of scientific knowledge to health problems, and an ethical component that demands the decision to be ethically justified" (Coughlin, 2009, p. 96).

To simplify the process of decision making in various situations, many authors propose models for solving dilemmas. However, most of these models involve, in some form or another, the same steps. Typically, making a decision starts with identifying the problem and then proceeds to gathering the relevant facts. Having done that, the person dealing with the problem lays out the alternative solutions, evaluates them, and then selects the most appropriate course of action. While acting to solve the problem, the person continues to evaluate the selected action to ensure its merits. An action that survives such evaluation is continued until the problem is resolved. These steps, which are adapted from several models, are summarized in Box 4-2. It is very important to also be able to determine which ethical principles are at stake and to apply ethical principles to the various options for solving the ethical dilemma.

Ethical dilemmas are usually solved in a similar way. For example, Darby and Walsh (2010) and Purtilo (1999) proposed schemes for solving ethical dilemmas that, in essence,

BOX 4-2

Decision-Making Steps

- Identify the problem: Define the problem or dilemma
- Gather the facts: Be a detective; ask questions
- List the alternatives: Brainstorm; list pros and cons
- Select the course of action: Justify the chosen action
- Act on the decision: Follow through on decision
- Evaluate the action: Judge the results of the action

simulate the previously mentioned steps. Their schemes, however, use specific terms that match the ethical context. For example, selecting the course of action is called "establishing an ethical position," and consulting theories of ethics are recommended for accomplishing this step. Purtilo recommends using normative ethical theories and taking into consideration the principles stressed by deontology, utilitarianism, and other ethical positions (see discussion in Chapter 1) while selecting a course of action. Rule and Veatch (2004) recommend also considering the ethical principles as found in professional codes of ethics. Specific decision-making steps are also found in the Code of Ethics of the CDHA (www.cdha.ca). An example of implementation of these eight steps are disussed by Neish and MacDonald (2003) in a ethical dilemma decision-making guide for solving an ethical dilemma.

At this point, it would be useful to reformulate the steps of decision making in a way that enables the dental hygienist to solve ethical dilemmas arising in daily practice. Box 4-3 offers an adaptation of the decision-making steps to guide solving ethical dilemmas facing dental hygienists:

BOX 4-3

Decision-Making Adaptation

- Gather the dental, medical, social, and all other clinically relevant facts of the case
- Identify all relevant values that play a role in the case and determine which values, if any, are in conflict
- List the options open to you to deal with the problem
- Choose the best solution from an ethical point of view
- Justify this solution
- Respond to possible criticism of the selected solution (Weinstein, 1993, p. 44)

APPLYING DECESION-MAKING STEPS

In this seection, each step will be considered as the chapter's case study is analyzed. Many of the steps overlap and flow into the next. Indentifying the problem should also identify the ehtical issue and what ethical principles are at stake. Likewise, selecting a course of actinon will involve jutifying and defending the decision based on ethical principles. The steps required for decision making may be further understood in light of the following explanations.

Identify the Problem

Before we can solve a problem, we need to know its dimensions and implications. There may not be a clear view; therefore, we need to determine what needs to be solved. This involves analyzing the problem and finding out whether it involves any violation of ethical principles. It is crucial to clearly determine whether there is an actual ethical dilemma, just a clash of personalities, or different interpretations of the issue. Thus, identifying the problem includes deciding whether the problem is an ethical dilemma. This is not always obvious. Good questions to ask are the following: Is it a matter of the way things are *done in the office* versus lack of *standard of care*, or is it a matter of following the Dental/Dental Hygiene Practice Act versus following a code of ethics? Is it a conflict between self-interest and acting morally? Can the ethical issues be identified?

DECISION-MAKING STEP #1 Referring to the case study at the beginning of the chapter, a decision needs to be made to:

- Follow the clinical protocol and not allow the family to return to the clinic.
- Ignore the rule and continue scheduling the family for dental treatment.
- Have the mother call when she is able to bring the children and schedule as many in as possible in between other patients' appointments.

Gather the Facts

There is an old axiom that says "Don't assume anything." In solving an ethical dilemma, it may be necessary to act as a detective, to ask the *what, when, where, why,* and *how* questions. We must also clarify assumptions and separate them from facts. Moreover, we must be aware of available sources of information about the relevant issue. In a study of dental students and how they would solve ethical dilemmas, it was found that students were not aware of certain avenues open to them. For example, in finding low-quality dental care in a new patient, dental students did not think of contacting a dental review board or a dentist who had done previous dental care on a patient (Bebeau et al., 1985). This shows the importance of understanding a profession's code of ethics, standards of care, professional liabilities, and legal regulations.

DECISION-MAKING STEP #2 Based on the information provided in the case study at the beginning of the chapter, the family does not keep the appointments. The mother does not work regularly scheduled hours and is the sole provider.

- She lives 45 minutes away. The mother does not receive appointment confirmation calls from the clinic to cancel the appointment because she does not have the minutes on her cell phone. And, she cannot receive calls at work.
- In the past, she has had the same problem with other Medicaid clinics, where there was a problem of missed appointments.

- The children are in great need of dental care and she is the only one who can take them to their appointments.
- By the children's not showing for appointments, other patients are not able to be seen during this time and the clinic is not able to have productive time to pay the dentist's salary.
- The ethical principle of beneficence, doing good for these children, is a factor. Another factor is justice or fairness, as other patients could be seen during this time.

List the Alternatives

It is always useful to have several possible solutions for a problem. Whenever there are many alternatives, a better solution is likely to be found. Brainstorming is enhanced by listing all reasonable suggestions rather than sticking to one or a few alternatives. Sometimes it is the suggestion that first appeared to be the most unlikely that eventually proves to be the best. However, we must exclude unreasonable alternatives as soon as it becomes clear that they are not going to help. Alternative solutions should take into consideration the concerns and obligations (both rights and duties and wants and needs) of all those involved in a situation. An alternative that ignores the interests or duties of one party is unlikely to be a reliable solution.

Sometimes an alternative seems warranted for one situation but not for others. This is why it is important to realize that solutions should be sensitive to the context. For example, it is generally improper to allow a dental assistant or dental hygienist to perform procedures not approved by the Dental/Dental Hygiene Practice Act. If you see a dental hygienist doing a procedure that the act assigns only to dentists, your list of alternatives would include advising the hygienist not to do so.

But suppose that a dental assistant or hygienist is very skilled at a procedure that is supposed to be done only by a dentist. You see him or her performing this procedure in a public facility in an underserved rural area where no dentist is available. If you think in terms of the nonmaleficence and utilitarian principles, you would probably find nothing wrong with that situation. Then you may include the choice of "turning a blind eye" to the situation among your list of alternatives. If you chose not to object to the violation of the act in that particular situation, you would be making a distinction between what is administratively or legally wrong and what is morally wrong. Indeed, what is legal and administratively correct is not always morally wrong and vice versa. However, conflicts between moral and legal judgments are likely to arise only in exceptional situations.

DECISION-MAKING STEP #3 In making decisions, one can always do nothing, that in itself is making a decision. However, many times one needs to do more than ignore the situation. In this chapter's case study, the decision needs to be make *to schedule* or *not to schedule* the children in the future.

1. The first alternative would be to do nothing.

The **pros** of this decision would be that there would be a chance that the family would be seen again and further treatment would be given.

The **cons** of this decision would be that clinic rules are not being followed and there would be a chance that this would happen again and, then, nothing would be solved, clinic would still be losing money, and other patients would not be able to be seen due to booking the time for this family.

2. The second alternative would be to enforce the clinic's rule and not to see the family again.

The **pros** of this decision would be that there would be no wasted appointment time nor loss of clinic income; thus, other patients could be booked, including emergency patients. The clinic would be adhering to established policies, and this decision would be a deterrent for other patients to *not show*.

The **cons** of this decision would be that the treatment would not be available to the family, including the children, which may lead to more serious health problems; additional administrative work would be needed to inform the mother that they are no longer patients.

3. The third alternative would be to bend the rules and allow the family to be seen.

The **pros** of this decision would be that the family would be seen. The mother would call when she has time off work and the clinic would attempt to schedule them at that time.

The **cons** of this decision would be that other patients would think that the *no-show* rule is not enforced and they may start to miss appointments; the family may miss more appointments; productive time would be lost for the clinic; and other patients could have been seen during that time. Other patients would just show up for unscheduled appointments. Also, once an exception is made for one family, others are entitled to similar expectations.

4. The fourth alternative would be to give the family another chance with stipulations. The mother would have to leave a phone number of a neighbor, friend, or relative where the clinic could call to inform the mother about the appointment time. However, the mother would also have to call back to confirm that she received the information and that she would keep the appointment. If she was not able to keep the appointment, she would have to give the clinic 24 hours' notice so that other patients could be booked during that time.

The **pros** of this decision would be that the children would have another chance to receive treatment. Also, the responsibility of confirming the appointment is given to the mother.

The **cons** of this decision would be that other patients may perceive this as special treatment.

Select the Course of Action

Having evaluated the alternatives, we need to select the course of action. This involves weighing the negative with the positive aspects of each possible course of action. The risks involved with each action also need to be identified. That is, we should ask the question: What could go wrong if a particular course of action is selected? At the same time, we should identify the merits of each possible course of action. Could that action be defended or justified on the grounds of moral principles and the values of the code of ethics? Such a question must be answered before endorsing a course of action. The reason that actions should be scrutinized at a moral level is that moral judgments should not be arbitrary.

DECISION-MAKING STEP #4   Make a choice among the available four alternatives. However, decisions can be amended according to changes in situations. One should keep all alternatives open to be ready for unexpected developments. Suppose it was decided to attempt alternative number four. The clinic would call someone other than the mother to inform her of the appointment, and she would call the clinic to confirm she received the message. If she is unable to keep the appointment, she will call the clinic at least 24 hours before the time of the appointment.

Act on the Decision

The aim of considering the alternatives and then assessing their advantages and disadvantages is to act in light of careful analysis of the situation. Acting becomes easy when we are sure that the selected action is justifiable. The best actions are those that survive ethical scrutiny. The consequences of such actions are often rewarding. Perhaps the least desirable consequence of morally justified actions is creating a conflict of interest. When we choose an action that runs against the preferences of superiors, there is always the risk of losing a job or friendships. Sometimes, worse consequences, such as losing reputation or status in the community, follow an action that may seem wrong to those who were not aware of all the aspects of the situation. However, we must act according to moral principles and bravely face the consequences. Fortunately, there are always principled people in every society who will defend good decisions and moral actions.

DECISION-MAKING STEP #5   Even though the selection of alternative number four may seem like special consideration, it seems the best solution in terms of the children receiving treatment and the clinic producing income. It would be based on the utilitarian principle and beneficence.

Evaluate the Action

In evaluating a selected action, a good question to ask is, if it happened again, would I make the same decision? A positive answer often implies the soundness of that action. We may also determine the effect of our decisions on the growth and development of the profession. Some good actions may initially look questionable but eventually lead to positive change in the practice of the profession. This is why we should continue to evaluate an action until all its consequences become clear. The implications of an action for ourselves, other members of the profession, and the community as a whole should be assessed. Actions that were previously evaluated and found satisfactory should be adopted, while actions that were not well received should be revised. The dental hygienist should welcome every critique and all feedback about a selected action.

DECISION-MAKING STEP #6   Yes, the clinic would do this again. It has worked well for the mother and the children. This alternative has also been used for other patients in similar situations where it has been a problem to confirm appointments resulting in *no-shows*. It also allows the patients to take more responsibility for confirming the appointments. The clinic is less likely to have lost productive time and more patients are actually being seen and receiving treatment. Using the case study, the clinic could revise the selected decision whenever problems for the clinic or the patients emerge. More decision should be flexible in the face of changeable reality.

In evaluating and reflecting on the decision or action, additional questions or *tests* can be asked. Chapdelain, Ruiz, Warchal, and Wells (2005) suggest one of the following tests: pillow, newspaper, or child. The specific questions are outlined in Box 4-4.

BOX 4-4

Testing the Decision

• Pillow test	Can you sleep with your decision?
• Newspaper test	Would you be comfortable having your decision published in the newspaper?
• Child test	Would you tell a child to engage in this behavior? (Or explain to a child the worthiness of the choice)

(Chapdelain, Ruiz, Warchal, & Wells, 2005, pp. 20, 33).

Summary

Throughout life, individuals are faced with both personal and professional decisions. An ethical dilemma occurs when there is a conflict between moral principles (refer to previous chapters). The capability to solve ethical dilemmas is acquired from the individual's progression through levels and stages of moral development. Other factors, such as age, education, gut feeling, and personality, may also determine solutions to ethical problems. Yet the awareness of moral principles and theories crucially enhances attaining this ability. There are several models of decision making, but the majority of them include identifying the problem, gathering the facts, listing the alternatives, selecting the course of action, acting, and evaluating the action.

Critical Thinking

1. Investigate decision-making models used by the authors to solve ethical dilemmas presented in dental and dental hygiene publications. Case scenarios are often included as an ongoing section or a featured item in the professional literature.
2. Create a case scenario based on your experience as a dental hygiene student. Solve the ethical dilemma, outlining each step of the solution. Share the decision-making process with a fellow student, a small group of students, or the class. What role did the ADHA, the CDHA, or IFDH Code of Ethics play in your decision making? What were the perceived obstacles to overcome for moral behavior, for a balance of good over harm, for patient autonomy, for justice and fairness, and for practicing within the legal boundaries of dental hygiene practice?
3. Write a one-page reaction to an ethical problem or issue discussed in one of the many case scenarios found in this textbook.
4. Explain how ethical dilemmas are different from other decision-making situations in your daily life.
5. Attempt to solve the case studies found in this textbook and MyHealthProfessionsKit using the steps found in Box 4-2. Defend the recommended action utilizing core values or ethical principles. Did the legal system or Dental/Dental Hygiene Practice Act play a role in determining the action to be taken?
6. In this chapter's case study, would you choose another alternative? How would you defend that decision?

Note: Case study for this chapter contributed by Teri McSherry, RDH, MSW. She is Assistant Instructor and Clinic Manager, Community Dental Center, Southern Illinois University Carbondale, IL.

CHAPTER 5

Jurisprudence

OBJECTIVES

After reading the material in this chapter, you will be able to

- Compare the concepts of civil law with criminal law, using examples found in dental hygiene practice.

- List the types and circumstances of *supervision* (or absence of supervision) found in the Dental/Dental Hygiene Practice Act of the jurisdiction (i.e., state, province, territory, or country) in which you reside or attend school, or where you would like to live or practice dental hygiene.

- State the conditions necessary for a contract between a patient and a dental hygienist with regard to dental hygiene services.

- Define and distinguish between the following terms:

  intentional tort and *unintentional* tort

  malpractice and *negligence*

  libel and *slander*

  assault and *battery*

  implied contract and *expressed* contract

- Discuss the *rights* of patients protected by law and *duties* of providers regulated by law from both *ethical* and *legal* perspectives.

- Discuss the role of lobbying in developing legislation for the practice of dental hygiene.

KEY TERMS

Abandon	Case law	Contracts
Accreditation	Certification	Contributory negligence
Assault	Civil law	Credentials
Battery	Common law	Criminal law

Defamation	Negligence	Standard of care
Forensic dentistry	Preceptorship	Standard negligence
Insurance fraud	Professional negligence	Statutory law
Jurisprudence	Risk management	Technical assault
Libel	Scope of practice	Technical battery
Lobbying	Self-regulation	Torts
Malpractice	Slander	

INTRODUCTION

In the practice of dental hygiene there are both ethical and legal considertions. In Chapter 3, we encountered confidentiality as both an ethical obligation and a legal obligation. This chapter will discuss some of the other legalities of dental hygiene pracitce, including clincial and administrative procedures. As a dental hygiene student, you may be preparing to write a national examination and to sit for a clinical examination which are necessary for licensure, a legal requirement to practice dental hygiene. As a dental hygienist you will also want to provide the best care possible for your patient and to prevent any danger of malpracitce. Finally, as a dental hygienist, you will want to further your profession using the legal system to enhance alternative pracitce settings.

Examples of laws found in dental hygiene practice are state dental practice acts, rules and regulations governing the practice of dental hygiene, discrimination laws, child abuse reporting, regulations of the Occupational Safety and Health Administration (OSHA), and insurance practices. There are a range of penalties for violation of laws, including administrative warnings (which amount only to reprimands), losses or suspensions of license, monetary or community service fines, mandatory education (either professional continuing education or social education), and prison sentences. Not knowing the law is not an excuse for not obeying the law. Thus, an introduction into jursiprudence is relevant.

Case Study

After leaving the employment of a dental office, you tell patients how your former supervisor/ employer dentist was not current in practice, that is, not keeping up to date in the field of dentistry and the delivery of oral health services. Although there was no actual harm to any patient, the dentist did not practice with a high standard of care. That was the main reason you left the office (i.e., the potential of harm). Your motive is not to have them switch to the new office, where you are currently working, but simply to inform them.

As you read this chapter, consider the following: Have you violated any ethical principles? Have you committed a crime or civil wrong?

CRIMINAL LAW

Jurisprudence is the science or philosophy of law (Hanks, 1986, p. 829), which may also include the establishment, regulation, and enforcement of legislation. **Statutory law** is enacted by legislation through U.S. Congress, state legislatures, or local legislative bodies (Miller & Hutton, 2000, p. 7).

TABLE 5-1   Comparison of Criminal Law and Civil Law

Context	Criminal Law	Civil Law
Initiator of legal action	Government (state, county, etc.)	Individual
Crime is against	Society	Individual
Agreement of jurors	Unanimous (all jurors)	51% (majority of jurors)
Payment of damages	Life, liberty, fine	Nominal, compensatory, punitive
Guilty of crime	Beyond a reasonable doubt	Responsible for the crime

The two types of statutory law are criminal law and civil law. **Criminal law** involves crimes against society or the public, with the government initiating legal action, and **civil law** involves crimes against an individual, with the harmed individual initiating the legal action.

Criminal law concerns offenses or wrongful acts against society and should protect the public's interest, whereas civil law concerns offenses or wrongful acts against an individual, including the individual's property and reputation. Additional comparisons between criminal law and civil law are found in Table 5-1. Criminal law seeks to punish the offender, while civil law seeks to compensate the victim (Davison, 2000, p. 34). Criminal law applies to everyone. For example, no matter who you are, it is wrong to kill or steal. In a criminal case, a jury must unanimously agree on a judgment, and the prosecutors, who represent society, must prove guilt beyond a reasonable doubt. If found guilty in a criminal case, an individual could lose life (death penalty) or liberty (prison sentence) or be fined (payment with either money or community service). It is important to recognize that there is overlap between civil and criminal laws because what affects an individual sometimes also affects the public and vice versa.

PURPOSE OF LICENSE   Performing dental hygiene procedures without having a license is a violation of criminal law. The purpose of a license is to protect the public. For example, the state government grants licensure to drive a car. To drive a car, an individual needs to obtain a driver's license to prove that he or she is able to obey the traffic laws and drive safely. This is to protect the public. If a person disobeys the law, he or she may be penalized with a jail term or a monetary or community service fine. Likewise, a dental hygienist must obtain a license from the state to ensure that he or she can safely provide specific treatment to the public. When the student has completed a recognized educational program and passed both a national written board examination and a practical examination, a state agency will grant a license to practice. If an individual practices dental hygiene without a license or performs procedures not allowed by the state dental practice act, he or she is performing a criminal act, and this may be considered a felony (Pollack & Marinelli, 1988, p. 30). An individual can be jailed or fined, or his or her dental hygiene license may be revoked or suspended for not complying with the guidelines of the state dental practice act, which is legislated law.

Insurance Fraud

Another criminal act that may be committed in dental hygiene practice is **insurance fraud**, which is intentional or deliberate misrepresentation for financial or personal gain. Examples in the dental office include inflating bills or falsifying billing costs for insurance reimbursement.

Other examples may include inaccurate dates of treatment and the nature of treatment actually provided. By participating in fraud, we may be helping the patient financially, but we are harming our personal integrity and the reputation of those we work with. In fact, insurance fraud is white-collar crime.

POST-DATING TREATMENT   A dental hygienist may be asked by a patient to postdate a treatment appointment. Frequently, insurance guidelines dictate that specific services may be performed only within a certain period. For example, preventive dental hygiene treatment will be reimbursed only every six months. Suppose a male college student was seen by the dental hygienist in early April during spring break and wants to schedule the next appointment before school starts in the fall. He asks the dental hygienist to postdate the appointment so that the insurance company pays for the treatment. Should the dental hygienist postdate the treatment to October and not September, fraud has occurred.

PRE-DATING TREATMENT   Likewise, predating treatment for insurance coverage is also fraud. A female college student, let us suppose, has graduated a month before her dental hygiene appointment and no longer has student health and dental insurance. If the dental hygienist stated that the treatment was done earlier to help this student avoid out-of-pocket payment, he or she is also committing insurance fraud. Other types of fraud (e.g., claiming that something was done when it was not done) may also occur in the dental hygiene employment environment as in any other work or personal situation.

ADDITIONAL TREATMENT   Claiming that additional work was in the treatment plan when that work was not really done is like claiming more damage on a car than actually occurred in an accident. A dental hygienist could be considered guilty of fraud in certain situations even though he or she may not have actually signed the insurance forms. If a dental hygienist is aware of a fraud committed by a patient or coworker and does not report it, he or she could be considered guilty by association. Again, this illegal fraudulent action would be tried in criminal court. It should be noted that patients can also be prosecuted for submitting fraudulent claims (Miller, 2006, p. 534).

CIVIL LAW

Two subsets of civil law are tort law and contract law. Civil law affects the dental hygiene practice when the dental hygienist does a procedure or fails to perform a procedure and the patient brings legal action against the dental hygienist. For example, if the dental hygienist caused harm while giving local anesthetic and it was illegal according to the Dental/Dental Hygiene Practice Act for a dental hygienist to administer local anesthetic, then there has been harm to society and to the individual. This involves both criminal and civil laws.

There are three types of damage that an individual who is found guilty in civil court can be ordered to pay. Box 5-1 lists the types of civil damages. The first type is *nominal*, or the actual cost of the damage, such as the cost of actually having a car repaired or a tooth restored. The second type is *compensatory* and includes nominal damages plus extra cost incurred. Compensatory damages are imposed to compensate for the nonmaterial and material harm caused to an individual. These damages may include lost wages or salary, pain and suffering, and medical expenses, whether present or future. The third type is *punitive* and goes beyond compensating the victim; it is imposed to punish the individual who is found responsible for harming a victim. Its idea is to

BOX 5-1

Types of Civil Damages

- Nominal   cost of damage
- Compensatory   compensate for harm
- Punitive   punish individual

deter others and to keep the perpetrator away from society to avoid further crimes. In health care, we may hear the expression "suing so one never practices again"—that would be punitive because it aims at an action that exceeds specific compensation.

TORT LAW

Two subsets of civil law that are of concern for the practice of dental hygiene are torts and contracts. **Torts** are civil wrongs. They can be either *intentional* or *unintentional*. In addition, they can be acts of *omission* (i.e., not doing something that should have been done) or acts of *commission* (i.e., doing something incorrectly). Examples of intentional torts in which there are intentions to harm are assault and battery, misrepresentation, defamation, and breach of confidentiality.

Professional Negligence and Malpractice

Negligence is an example of an unintentional tort; a dental hygienist did not intend to harm the patient, but his or her action or inaction inflicted harm. **Negligence** is the failure to perform a clinical action (prophylactic or therapeutic) at the reasonable and acceptable standards of the profession with the result of harm to the patient. A mistake *without* harm does not constitute negligence. In dental hygiene practice, negligence may be an act of omission or commission. Both are considered negligence.

- **Professional negligence** is neglecting to perform a procedure or action that is part of standard of care—that is, doing or failing to do what a reasonable and prudent dental hygienist would do under the same circumstances. It may occur at any time during the various stages of patient care, including during assessment, treatment, and follow-up.
- **Standard negligence**, or ordinary negligence, does not involve patient care. According to Scott (2000), if a patient falls on a slippery floor in a hospital and is harmed, ordinary negligence is involved since falling on a slippery floor can happen anywhere—inside or outside a hospital—and does not involve direct patient care.

Case Study Follow-up #1

Is the dentist being negligent by not keeping up in dentistry?

Is the dentist guilty of malpractice?

TESTIMONY   Professional negligence may be substantiated by an *expert witness*. An expert witness is someone who is highly knowledgeable in a specialized area. For example, if a dental hygienist was accused of not following standard precautions, an expert witness could be a representative from OSHA or a dental professional who publishes or teaches in the area of bloodborne pathogens. The testimony, a statement of truth or fact, of this expert witness could defend the actions of the *defendant* (the dental hygienist accused of causing harm) by stating that the appropriate measures and standard of care were used. The expert witness could also testify against the dental hygienist and speak on behalf of the *plaintiff* (the patient who was harmed and is suing for professional negligence) and declare that appropriate measures and standard of care were not used. In the case of the slippery floor, one does not need an expert to determine that the floor was slippery. Ordinary eyewitnesses can attest to whether it was slippery.

EVIDENCE   In some cases of professional negligence, an expert witness may not be needed. The evidence is presented under the doctrine of *res ipsa loquitur* (the thing speaks for itself). This would occur, for example, if an instrument tip broke and was left in the sulcus or if treatment was performed on the wrong tooth. In other lawsuits, evidence can be judged from what is presented, or *prima facie* (at first sight). At times, a patient may contribute to the negligence or harm; this is referred to as **contributory negligence**. The patient has not taken reasonable care to protect his or her safety and thus has *contributed* to the injury or harm. For example, a patient may not take prophylactic pre-medication as instructed before a procedure. The dental hygienist who treats a patient without asking if the premedication was taken is considered negligent. However, the patient has also contributed to negligence by not following the instructions. If harm results from not being premedicated, the dental hygienist is considered negligent, but the patient is also held contributory to negligence. This can be an important legal defense for a dental hygienist whose patient was noncompliant with recommendations (Davison, 2000, p. 51).

Professional negligence that causes *harm* is **malpractice** (bad practice). For malpractice to occur, it must be established that an individual, a patient, was actually *harmed* because of a lack of standard of care. The minimal level of care that is recognized by a professional group as appropriate is **standard of care**. For example, treating a patient who needs prophylactic coverage with antibiotics without the proper premedication is in itself not malpractice as long as no harm occurred. However, failure to premedicate a patient who needs antibiotic coverage, resulting in that patient developing infective endocarditis or hematogenous total joint infection (diffuse hematogenous joint infection), is malpractice. Harm has resulted from not premedicating a patient at risk, which is failure to meet the standard of care for a patient who needs antibiotics before dental hygiene treatment. This standard of care is recommended by the American Dental Association, the American Heart Association, and the American Academy of Orthopedic Surgeons (Daniel, Harfst, & Wilder, 2008, p. 241).

There are three conditions necessary to prove malpractice as outlined in Box 5-2. It should be understood that dental hygienists have a duty to deliver standard of care to avoid the charge of malpractice.

ENSURING STANDARD OF CARE   Causes of malpractice include ignorance, lack of skill, neglect in applying skills, professional misconduct, lack of fidelity in performance of professional duties, and practice contrary to established rules. Therefore, dental hygienists must ensure that they give a high quality of care. Among the means of achieving this aim are continuing education courses, cardiopulmonary resuscitation (CPR) certification, using critical-thinking skills in judgments regarding patient care, and being always aware of the standards of care in one's

---

BOX 5-2

Conditions of Malpractice

The conditions of malpractice are the following:

- There was an act of omission or commission
- There was failure to satisfy standard of care
- There was harm or injury to the patient

---

locale. Most important, dental hygienists should know when to refer a patient to the appropriate expert because we cannot all be experts. In addition, dental hygienists may need to make decisions regarding patient care if their standard of care differs from the standards of others involved in the treatment of patients, such as dentists. Standards of practice including competencies have been developed by the American Dental Education Association (www.sdea.org), American Dental Hygienists' Association (www.adha.org) and the Canadian Dental Hygienists Association (www.cdha.ca).

COMMUNICATION   Malpractice cases could often be avoided through better communication between the provider and the patient. Good communication can often prevent court cases when the outcome of treatment was not what the patient expected. Following the protocols of informed consent and the patient as a partner model (as discussed in Chapter 3) may prevent a patient from suing. Informed consent is both ethical and legal. Paige (1977) cites two reasons for suing: unreasonable patient expectations and impersonal care (e.g., provider showing no interest). Likewise, Miller (2006) suggests that "health care providers who maintain good relationships with their patients before and after incidents are less likely to be sued" (p. 588). Accusations of malpractice can be avoided by resolving disputes internally and early, maintaining a dialogue with patients, practicing quality record keeping, being open to offering a refund, and referring early in treatment to a more experienced specialist (Curley, 1997, p. 24).

PREVENTING NEGLIGENCE   Although the majority of dental hygienists work under the supervision of dentists, they may be charged with negligence. An example of negligence on the part of the dental hygienist would be failing to inform the patient, the dentist, or both about periodontal condition (Paige, 1977, p. 167). Negligence could also be charged if the dental hygienist did not provide standard of care, such as by not following the standard precaution protocol, with the result of causing disease transmission. Failure to probe that leads to undetected periodontal disease is another example of negligence. Under the principle *respondeat superior*, the dentist, as employer and supervisor, may also be responsible for the actions of the dental hygienist. But this does not relieve the dental hygienist from the guilt of neglect. Even though the dentist may be accountable for the actions of a dental hygienist, the latter may still be named as codefendant. Thus, it is very important that dental hygienists have their own malpractice insurance (this will be further discussed in Chapter 11).

Assault and Battery

Assault and battery are other examples of *torts*, or civil wrongs, and may be considered in either criminal or civil court. **Assault** is threatening to harm an individual. **Battery** is touching an individual with the intention to harm. **Technical assault** or **technical battery** may occur even in the absence of the intention to harm if there is no permission to touch. For example, attempting to perform or actually performing treatment that the patient did not consent to is technical assault or technical battery. The terms may be used interchangeably. For example, applying a desensitizing agent to a tooth or a topical anesthetic to gingival tissue may be considered technical battery if the patient was not informed that this may be part of dental hygiene debridement therapy although the intent is to make the patient feel more comfortable. A good rule is to always tell the patients what you are doing and why, so that they can agree to each procedure. What may seem a routine act to the clinician may not seem routine to patients. This is why patients expect and deserve informative explanations.

Accusations of technical assault or technical battery can be avoided by obtaining informed consent. In our example, the patient did not give implied or expressed consent to topical anesthesia. The patient can argue that he or she gave no authorization to perform a procedure that was not mentioned. In that case, giving topical anesthesia without prior consent amounts to assault. The situation would be even worse for the dental hygienist if the topical anesthetic caused an adverse reaction, the possibility of which the patient was not informed of in advance. However, some states may consider lack of informed consent disclosure as negligence or malpractice and not as assault and battery (Litch & Liggett, 1992; Rossoff, 1981).

Defamation

A third possible tort that may occur in dental hygiene practice is defamation. **Defamation** is making false statements that harm an individual's reputation and involves communication to a third person. Criticizing the treatment provided by another dental hygienist directly to that dental hygienist is not defamation. However, falsely criticizing the treatment provided by another dental hygienist to someone else (e.g., another dental hygienist, a dentist, or a patient) is defamation. There are two types of defamation. **Libel** is written or published defamation. **Slander** is oral defamation. Although it is unethical to criticize another professional's care to a patient, it may also be a *civil* wrong if the criticism is untrue.

Frequently, dental hygienists may be in a position to criticize the standard of care given to patients provided by another dental hygienist or dentist. However, we need to be cautious, as we do not know the circumstance in which the care was given and to what degree the patient may have contributed to the alleged negligence. Perhaps the patient never returned for follow-up appointments, or the dental hygienist faced problems beyond his or her control. In addition to written and oral false statements, defamation may also occur with the inappropriate release of inaccurate medical information (e.g., patients' charts). Knowing that there is no foundation for what is being said about a patient and saying it anyway is fraud. There has been intentional misrepresentation and harm could occur (Pozgar, 1996, p. 71).

Case Study Follow-up #2

Has the dental hygienist committed slander?

Has the dental hygienist acted ethically by "warning" her patients?

BOX 5-3

Types of Contracts

- Implied (assumed)
- Expressed (either oral or written)

CONTRACT LAW

Contracts are agreements and obligations. The two types of contracts are implied and expressed (see Box 5-3). *Implied* contracts are assumed contracts; the parties need not have discussed the agreement in detail but have shown interest in making a contract. For example, a patient sitting in the dental hygienist's chair and the dental hygienist providing treatment shows an interest in a contract between the dental hygienist and the patient; the patient will receive treatment, and the dental hygienist will give treatment. *Expressed* contracts are orally stated or written agreements by the involved parties.

CONDITIONS OF A CONTRACT   Courts have found that even a phone conversation between a provider and a patient constitutes a contract. Care plans are good examples of expressed contracts. Situations that legally require written consent include trying new drugs, experimenting with new procedures, taking a patient's photograph, giving general anesthesia, treating minor children in public programs, and providing treatment for more than one year. It may be helpful to review Chapter 3 and informed consent. Box 5-4 lists the conditions of a contract.

Contracts are binding under three conditions: (1) the parties must be competent, (2) specific acts must be mutually agreed on, and (3) there is a promise of something (i.e., payment for dental hygiene procedures) in return for something else (i.e., dental hygiene services). A patient arriving for a dental hygiene appointment is giving consent or agreement to have dental hygiene therapy. The agreement is usually that the dental hygienist will provide specific treatment and that the patient will pay for these dental hygiene services. Conditions for breach of contract are described in Box 5-5.

BOX 5-4

Conditions of a Contract

- Competency
- Specific acts must be mutually agreed
- Something in return for something else

BOX 5-5

Conditions for Breach of Contract

- Rights have been violated
- Services not performed
- Services are delayed

In dental hygiene, a *breach of contract* occurs when (1) financial rights or privacy rights have been violated, (2) services agreed to are not performed, or (3) services are delayed for an extended period. Harm *does not* have to occur for there to be a breach of contract. Under contract law, the dental hygienist, as a health care provider, has duties to the patient. These duties are outlined in Box 5-6. As you can see, many of the duties to a patient considered in a legal contract are also within the domain of acting ethically and following the Code of Ethics of the American Dental Hygienists' Association (ADHA), the Canadian Dental Hygienists Association (CDHA), or the Internatioan Federation of Dental Hygienists (IFDH). Many of these duties, such as keeping accurate records and other legal documents, will be covered further in this chapter and future chapters, as well as MyHealthProfessionsKit.

BOX 5-6

Duties of a Dental Hygienist as a Health Care Provider

- To provide standard of care
- To be licensed
- To obtain informed consent
- To keep current with treatment modalities
- To render treatment within a reasonable time
- To refer when necessary
- To charge a reasonable fee
- To treat within the scope of practice
- To keep accurate records
- To achieve a reasonable therapeutic or clinical result
- To provide patient instructions
- To inform patient of unexpected occurrences
- To maintain confidentiality
- To not abandon the patient
- To observe the fiduciary relationship created with the patient to maintain trust
- To exercise reasonable skill, care, and judgment in diagnosis and treatment

BOX 5-7

Duties of a Patient as a Health Care Partner

- Providing accurate and complete information about their complaint and health history and reporting any changes in their conditions (e.g., pain, effects of medications, and other drugs they are taking)
- Following the recommendations and instructions regarding treatment that they accepted
- Fulfilling financial obligations as much as possible (e.g., paying bills and reporting changes with insurance companies)
- Keeping appointments or making timely cancellations or rescheduling of appointments
- Respecting the rights of other patients and their companions, health care providers, personnel associated with the delivery of treatment, and other staff members

PATIENTS AS PARTNERS   Duties owed to the patient can be found in codes of ethics, practice acts, patients' bill of rights, and other documents. What about patient duties owed to caregivers and health care providers? As partners in their own care, patients should seek detailed information about their conditions and ask questions when they need to be more informed. Patients also should be responsible for adopting lifestyles that affect their health. Other duties on the part of the patients are listed in Box 5-7.

Abandonment

One of the duties of the provider is nonabandonment, except in specific situations allowed by law. A health care provider cannot **abandon** a patient, that is, terminate treatment or refrain from seeing the patient, unless certain criteria are met. These conditions are found in Box 5-8.

BOX 5-8

Legal Termination, Non-abandonment

The provider–patient relationship can be *legally* terminated if:

- Care is no longer needed (cured or treatment completed)
- Patient withdraws from the relationship,
- Care of the patient is transferred to another health care provider
- Ample notice of withdrawal is given
- Provider is unable to provide care (e.g., because of death or not having the skill)
- Provider unilaterally decides to terminate care
- Both parties (patient and provider) agree to end it

(Darby & Walsh, 2010, p. 1194; Miller & Hutton, 2000, pp. 422–423).

In dental hygiene practice, a patient may be refused an appointment for a variety of reasons, such as repeated last-minute cancellations, not arriving for scheduled appointments, or noncompliance with home care. Nonpayment for services can be a valid reason for ending a relationship (Dietz, 2000, p. 57). However, it is recommended that the health care professional complete all treatment started even if the patient is not paying for services and that he or she continue follow-up care of the patient until the threat of postoperative complications has passed (Daniel, Harfst, & Wilder, 2008, p. 48; Davison, 2000, pp. 80–81).

TERMINATION PROCEDURE   To legally terminate the dentist/dental hygienist–patient relationship, certain steps must be followed to prevent the liability of abandonment. These are:

1. The patient has to be told *in writing* that the dentist or dental hygienist is terminating the relationship.
2. The letter should provide the reasons for the termination.
3. The letter should clarify that a copy of the patient's file will be sent to another dentist or dental hygienist on written and signed request.
4. The letter should be sent by certified or registered mail with a return receipt requested; both the letter and returned receipt should be kept in the patient's file.
5. The letter should contain a list of other providers of dental or dental hygiene care.
6. The letter should inform the patient of any further treatment needs to be performed by the prospective providers.
7. The patient must be given a sufficient time (e.g., 30 days or more) to locate another dentist or dental hygienist to provide treatment. During this transitional period, emergency treatment must be rendered when needed.

EXAMPLE   Abandonment can also occur if the health care provider does not arrange for coverage during absence. It is essential that a dentist or dental hygienist provide information about how to seek help during his or her absence. For example, the dental office may have a phone message on the answering machine that directs a patient to call a certain number in case of emergency (e.g., gives dentist's home/cell number or directs the patient to call another dentist or seek treatment at a specific facility). In addition, the provider should inform the patient about where to seek care if there is a planned absence (e.g., vacation or hospitalization) shortly after procedures that may need emergency follow-up treatment, such as after periodontal surgery or tooth extraction.

Risk Management

The actions taken to prevent financial loss or possible legal actions are referred to as **risk management**. Scott (2000) defines risk management as "the process of systematically monitoring health care delivery activities in order to prevent or minimize financial losses from claims or lawsuits arising from patient care or other activities conducted in a health care facility" (p. 191). In fact, risk-management approaches can actually improve quality of care by reviewing clinical procedures and protocols (Shi & Singh, 2010, p. 295). Two basic areas of risk management in the dental office are record keeping (i.e., good documentation) and informed consent (Bressman, 1993, p. 63). Dental hygienists can avoid court cases by knowing the law and applying it. Ignorance of the law *does not* render one immune to it.

DOCUMENTATION   In addition to good communication, the best protection from lawsuits is documentation. Records should be dated, signed, legible, and written in black or blue ink.

BOX 5-9

Elements of Good Documentation

- Identification of the problem
- Description of the procedure performed
- Notation of the level of involvement
- Evaluation of outcome

(Eubanks, 1992; Vaughn, 2007, p. 39).

Mistakes should never be whited out but crossed out with a single line, an explanation should be given for the change, the correct information should be given, initialed or signed, and dated (Miller, 2006, p. 436). Watterson (2010) advises that anyone who reads a patient's chart should be able to:

- Know what treatment the patient has had and why
- Perform whatever treatment is next for that individual and know why it is necessary (p. 52)

Elements of good documentation can be found in Box 5-9. In a court case, it is the defendant (i.e., the provider or dental hygienist) who needs to prove the absence of guilt. Individual states have laws regarding the length of time required for keeping records (e.g., 7 or 10 years). In addition, there are laws regarding the statute of limitations, that is, the length of time after an injury or damage (or when discovered) in which a patient can sue or file a lawsuit.

PREVENTION   Continuing education promotes risk management by providing up-to-date information regarding laws, standard of care, treatments, and clinical techniques (Healthcare Providers Service Organization, 2004). Cady (2009) states that the best defense is to assess, diagnose, and prescribe (p. 23). Others recommend taking risk management steps (see Box 5-10) through better teamwork in the dental office or other workplace.

BOX 5-10

Risk Management/Teamwork Steps

- Smart hires
- Communicate with clarity
- Evaluate effectively

(Vaughn & Harvey, 2008, pp. 42–44).

CASE LAW

Another type of law is **common law**, or **case law**, formulated by judges or determined by court decisions; common law is issued through judgments, *not* by legislation. For example, according to common law, some couples may be considered legally married after a given number of years of living together. Scott (1998) states that laws related to health care legal and ethical issues, business relationships among health professions and organizations, and most American civil legal authority derive from common law (p. 7). It is important to note that "common law can be changed by statues that modify the principles or by court decisions that establish different common law principles" (Miller, 2006, p. 13).

LICENSURE

The purpose of a license is to protect the public. A license can also be part of the evolution of an occupation and to grant it professional status. Thus, dental hygiene can be considered a profession because a license is needed to practice. In the United States, licensure or regulation of dental hygienists is determined by each state, in Canada by each province, and elsewhere by each country. The major method of licensure is through a government agency. Box 5-11 lists the members of the International Federation of Dental Hygienists. Of these members, dental hygiene practice is not regulated in Austria, Germany, and Slovakia (Johnson, 2009, p. 69).

Educational Requirements

As stated earlier, licensure is a government regulation. Usually, licensing laws have educational and examination requirements. An individual must graduate from an accredited dental hygiene program to be licensed (except in Alabama). **Accreditation** status means that the program has met the minimal requirement standards outlined by the Commission on Dental Accreditation of the American Dental Association (ADA) or the Commission on Dental Accreditation of the Canadian Dental Association (CDA). In member countries of the IFDH, graduation from an approved dental hygiene program is necessary (Johnson, 2009, p. 69).

EVALUATIVE MEASURES   These standards cover all phases of a dental hygiene program, including how students are admitted to patient confidentiality, and judge not only the academic

BOX 5-11

IFDH Membership

Australia	Finland	Japan	New Zealand	Spain
Austria	Germany	Korea	Norway	Sweden
Canada	Ireland	Latvia	Portugal	Switzerland
Denmark	Israel	Lithuania	Slovak Republic/Slovakia	United Kingdom
Fiji	Italy	Netherlands	South Africa	United States

component of the curriculum but also other aspects that influence the curriculum, including faculty, facilities, and finances. The areas evaluated are (1) institutional effectiveness; (2) educational program; (3) administration, faculty, and staff; (4) educational support services; (5) health and safety provisions; and (6) patient care (Commission on Dental Accreditation, 2007). Through accreditation, dental hygienists and the public are guaranteed that minimal educational standards are met for the practicing dental hygienist. Although dental hygienists may participate in accreditation site visits to dental hygiene programs, the dentists still control the education of dental hygienists because programs are accredited by the national dental associations (ADA or CDA) and not by the dental hygiene associations (ADHA or CDHA).

PRECEPTORSHIP   The majority of dental hygienists in North America are educated in community colleges and receive associate degrees; however, both the ADHA and the CDHA recommend that the baccalaureate be the entry-to-practice degree. Currently, Alabama is the only state that allows educational requirements to be attained through **preceptorship**, or on-the-job training. Dental hygiene preceptorship is the training of dental hygienists in the dental office by a dentist. Although there may be some official classroom requirements, such as basic sciences and clinical lectures, preceptor programs are not housed in an institution of higher learning. A dentist in Alabama is able to train an individual in a private dental office to be a dental hygienist with no standardized preclinical or clinical instruction, but there is a required number of patients to be treated and criteria for the mastery of skills (Curran & Darby, 1990, p. 293). However, both the dentist and the student have guidelines to follow regarding education requirements set forth by the Board of Dental Examiners of Alabama (2009).

Written Board Exams

One must have graduated (or will graduate within a certain period) from an accredited dental hygiene program to be eligible to take the National Board Dental Hygiene Examination. The Joint Commission on National Dental Examination is the agency responsible for the development and administration of the National Board Dental Hygiene Examination. This commission includes representatives from dental schools, dental practice, state dental examining boards, dental hygiene, and the public. In addition, a standing committee of the joint commission includes dental hygienists who act as consultants. For example, faculty of dental hygiene programs act as experts in specific content areas for the formulation of questions for test construction. This exam is a computer-written evaluation of theoretical knowledge through recall and case-based multiple-choice questions.

Likewise, in Canada, dental hygienists pass the National Dental Hygiene Certification Examination (NDHCE), the written exam of the National Dental Hygiene Certification Board. This exam is given in either English or French depending on the province or area of residence and practice. One striking difference between these two national board examinations is that in Canada dental hygienists have more control over the exam, whereas in the United States dentists (through the ADA) have more control. Globally, dental hygienists may need to take either a written exam, a clinical (practical) board or exam, or both.

Practical Board Exams

In addition to a written exam, dental hygienists may also be required to take a practical board exam. In this exam, dental hygienists are required to demonstrate competency in providing dental hygiene services such as recording medical histories, performing an oral examination, charting existing oral conditions, taking radiographs, probing, detecting and removing calculus, and polishing. There are differences among jurisdictions in the content of board exams, and each state or province may vary in terms of the passing score necessary. For example, the North East Regional Board Exam contains not only a patient treatment portion but also a computer-simulated exam portion, called the computer-simulated clinical exercise. It is taken via a computer that displays slides illustrating various clinical topics and clinical situations. For example, the candidate may be asked to name an anatomy structure found on a radiograph.

REGIONAL BOARDS   Alternatively, a state may elect to participate with a group of neighboring states and recognize a regional board exam. In the case of regional board exams, states contract with nonregulatory testing agencies or for-profit testing services to administer clinical examinations. In the United States, the regional board exams are North East Regional, Central Regional, Southern Regional, and Western Regional. Information regarding these board exams is found in MyHealthProfessionsKit.

Other Requirements for Licensure

As a student, you will decide where you plan to practice and take the practical board exam necessary for your state. Requirements for licensure are in a constant state of flux, and what was a requirement when you started dental hygiene may not be required now. Unfortunately, there are reciprocity restrictions. That is, although the national written board is recognized throughout the United States, practical boards are not. If a practicing dental hygienist moves from one state to another, there is no automatic transfer of license. For example, a dental hygienist who wants to practice in California needs to take the California board exam even though he or she is licensed in Illinois through one of the regional boards. In addition, the dental hygienist who moves to California is required to take an examination (with proof of required education) for local anesthesia, which is a legal function for dental hygienists in California but not in every state.

Although an individual state may recognize a regional board, it may have additional requirements for licensure, such as an examination covering the state dental practice act, continuing education courses in a specific area (e.g., child abuse, OSHA, or nitrous oxide), or CPR certification. Dental hygiene, along with dentistry, is one of the few professions that require practical examination as well as written examination. For example, nurses pass a national theory exam but do not need to take a practical exam. That is, they are not tested on nursing procedures such as taking blood pressure or changing a dressing. Some feel that this restriction on portability (relocation from state to state) is meant to protect the public, while others feel that it is meant to financially protect those in the field by preventing an oversupply to an area. Yet others feel that it is a way that one profession, dentistry, can have control over another profession, dental hygiene.

According to Richardson (2004), Canadian dental hygienists, the majority of which are self-regulating, have attained mobility from province to province (or jurisdiction to jurisdiction) through the Federation of Dental Hygiene Regulatory Authorities (formed by registrars or agencies that grant licensure or certification to practice dental hygiene) and a mutual recognition agreement under Canada's internal trade. **Self-regulation** means that dental hygienists oversee the practice of dental hygiene (they regulate themselves) and work directly with the government—and not through dentists—for licensing and other issues related to dental hygiene practice.

According to the Canadian Dental Hygienists Association (2010), all the provinces have achieved self-regulation with the exception of Prince Edward Island.

Although each province or territory is responsible for licensure or registration, the two basic requirements are graduation from an accredited program and the written exam (NDHCE). A province or jurisdiction may request additional competencies, such as expanded functions. In these situations, a temporary or limited certification (or license) may be given until the dental hygienist is able to attain the required skill or education (Richardson, 2004, p. 20). It would seem that self-regulation has granted dental hygiene in Canada more responsibility and at the same time eased the restrictions imposed on dental hygienists who wish to practice in other areas than where they were first licensed or received their dental hygiene education.

Outside of the United States and Canada, licensure is national and there is reciprocity between Australia and New Zealand, and with countries in the European Community. However, that is not the case everywhere. There have been discussions for the United States to have one national licensing exam and acceptance of education from outside countries (Givens, 2009; Fernandes, 2009; Richardson, 2004; Johnson, 2009).

Credentialing

Another way to receive a license is through **credentials**, or credentialing. Credentialing is determined by each state. Usually, dental hygienists practicing specific procedures prior to the introduction of exams or license for those procedures are recognized as competent. These dental hygienists are "grandfathered" into the profession or recognized with the ability to perform specific procedures based on prior experience or education. Licensure is granted on the basis of *the past* and not on the new regulations for licensure. Another way to credential is to document that the dental hygienist is equal in skills to those presently licensed. For example, a dental hygienist licensed in Ohio for many years may be granted a license in Illinois without additional examination requirements.

LICENSING METHODS   The grounds for granting credentials may include a dental hygiene employment history signed by former employers or supervising dentists, a dental hygiene diploma, national board exam results, an active license elsewhere, good standing with other dental hygiene licensing agencies, and continuing education credits. Individual state dental practice acts usually have a section regarding reciprocity and credentialing. An example of working definitions for licensure methods are found in Box 5-12.

Certification

A term often confused with licensing is **certification**. As already stated, the government grants license. Not all dental hygienists who are licensed are certified. Certification is granted by a nongovernmental entity, such as an organization, institution, agency, or association. For example, dental hygienists may take an expanded function course (e.g., restorative, orthodontic, local anesthesia, or nitrous oxide sedation). The certification is recognition that the dental hygienist had advanced training to perform these duties but not the license to perform these duties.

PRACTICE ACT

The state dental practice act is statutory law, passed by legislatures, that controls the practice of dentistry and dental hygiene; similarly, the provincial (or a jurisdiction) government is responsible for the practice of dental hygiene. Throughout the world, for the most part, dental hygiene

BOX 5-12

Licensure Methods and Definitions

• Examination	Applicant has applied for is required to take and pass all or a portion of an exam.
• Endorsement of license	Original license issued in another state and that state's requirements were substantially equivalent.
• Acceptance of Examination	Applicant has taken a national exam in any state; applicant may or may not be licensed in another state.
• Restoration	Applicant has previously been licensed in state and has allowed license to laps long enough to require reapplication; possible exam passage and/or committee review.
• Grandfather/Waiver	Applicant will be licensed without regard to current requirement because state allows this based on past qualifications and practice; may be for a specified time only.
• Nonexamination	Applicant is licensed by meeting qualifications required by statue; there is not an exam.

Adapted: Illinois Dental Practice Act (2006).

has a scope of practice. This legislation outlines the rules and regulations as interpretations of the law. In the state or provincial dental/dental hygiene practice act, procedures are stated in regards to what a dental hygienist can and cannot do. These may be a "laundry list" of itemized procedures, or the act may use general statements that define the procedures that dental hygienists may perform (e.g., preventive services) and those procedures reserved for only dentists (e.g., diagnosis). The act also sets forth the educational requirements for dental hygienists, including continuing education.

Protection

The purpose of the state or provincial dental/dental hygiene practice act is to protect the public, and depending on how the act is written and interpreted, it may also protect dentists and dental hygienists. Because the act is a law, it means that only those who abide by the act will be able to *legally* practice dental hygiene. Thus, unqualified personnel are prevented from jeopardizing the health of the consumer. In the past, copies of the act were hard to obtain, and some states charged a fee for copies. However, now each state's dental practice act is accessible on the Internet and you can download it. You will find links to each state's act at www.adha.org and www.ada.org, and links to Canadian practice information can be found at www.cdha.ca. Links can also be found at MyHealthProfessionsKit.

Regulation

The dental profession regulates the majority of dental hygienists in the United States through dental boards. Members of these boards are appointed by the governor and may consist of dentists, dental hygienists, consumers, and other members of the dental team. In the past, dental hygienists did not have voting rights on some dental boards. Dental hygienists are now viewed as equal members on these boards, although in many instances they are still outnumbered by dentists. New Mexico and Washington are two states that have self-regulation; that is, dental hygienists have authority in the regulation of dental hygiene. Other states have dental hygiene committees that make recommendations to the dental board. In addition, some states work with another nondental agency to regulate dentistry and dental hygiene. For example, in Illinois, the Department of Professional Regulations actually grants the license to practice dentistry and dental hygiene. Regulatory information on individual states can be obtained from the ADHA, ADA, and individual state dental and dental hygiene associations.

SELF-REGULATION IN CANADA   As stated earlier in this chapter, the majority of dental hygienists in Canada are *self-regulated*. Self-regulation began in Quebec in 1975 and spread to the larger provinces. The other provinces that are self-regulated are Alberta (which gained self-regulation in 1990), Ontario in 1993, British Columbia in 1995, and Saskatchewan in 1998 (Richardson, 2004, p. 18). Manitoba, Nova Scotia, and New Brunswick also have it. In June 2010, CDHA announced that Newfoundland and Labrador dental hygienists had attained self-regulation. Within twenty years (1990–2010), dental hygienists throughout Canada, with the exception of Prince Edward Island, have achieved self-regulation. Thus, dental hygienists in Canada, through self-regulation, are making progress in being recognized as a profession and not under the control of another profession (dentistry) whose members (dentists) are also the primary employers.

INTERNATIONAL REGULATION   As in the United States and Canada, dental hygienists must graduate from an approved dental hygiene program and take a written and/or clinical board examination. As stated earlier, dental hygienists in Austria, Germany, and Slovakia are not regulated. Australia, Ireland and New Zealand are regulated similarly to the United States, that is, by governing board consisting of mainly (if not entirely) of dentists. Latvia and South Africa have self-regulation. The other members of IFDH are regulated by government agencies such as departments of health (Johnson, 2009, p. 69).

U.S. LEGISLATIVE BILL   In the United States, changes in state dental practice acts are also made by legislation and are introduced as a bill. Then, according to legislative measures, a bill must be passed in both the state assembly and the state senate, either of which can stop a bill or amend it. A bill can also be sent to a specially formed committee to modify the areas of disagreement between the assembly and the senate and is again reviewed by both. If the bill passes, it is given to the governor to either sign or veto. Canadian dental hygienists, in comparison to U.S. dental hygienists, have their rules of practice determined by provincial legislation and ministries of health.

LOBBYING   The bill can also become a law without the governor's signature, although it is preferable to have this. It is important during the time a bill is being considered that dental hygienists lobby to get it passed. For example, if a proposed bill would transfer some dental hygiene functions to a less qualified group of practitioners, and dental hygienists disagree with that bill, we should contact the legislators to express our concerns. Dental hygienists should resist any attempt by any other group working in the dental field to take over functions from dental hygienists since that may jeopardize the dental hygiene profession.

Legislators can be contacted by individuals or through a dental hygiene association. It is useful for the dental hygiene profession to employ lobbyists who can effectively contact legislators and persuade them to vote a certain way—a way that ensures protecting the public as well as the interests of the dental hygiene profession. Dental hygienists can also participate in **lobbying** through activities such as writing editorials and informative articles in newspapers, meeting face-to-face with legislators, and working on legislators' campaigns to establish links with them. Being politically alert and active is essential for protecting the rights of the dental hygiene profession. More information on lobbying is in the Advocacy section of Chapter 6.

Scope of Practice

Most state or provincial dental/dental hygiene practice acts have a list of functions that dental hygienists can perform, referred to as a **scope of practice**. The scope of practice may also indicate procedures that the dental hygienist cannot perform. Some dental hygienists feel that an official list is restrictive to dental hygiene and implies that dental hygienists cannot do those procedures not specified in the list. Others feel that the list protects dental hygienists because it entails that no other dental team member is allowed to perform the functions allocated for dental hygienists. Some states have *open provisions* that allow the dentist to determine which functions dental hygienists can perform. In these circumstances, the dental hygienists are usually not allowed to perform those functions reserved for dentists, such as diagnosis, cutting tissue, and writing prescriptions (Davison, 2000, p. 105).

Supervision

Dental hygiene is one of the few professions that require supervision from another profession. In fact, supervision is one of the features that prevent dental hygiene from being recognized as a full (or true) profession by some individuals and various organizations. A few states (e.g., California and Colorado; and more recently, Maine) allow independent or unsupervised practice; however, specific functions need supervision by a dentist. For example, in Colorado, a dentist's physical presence is required for the administration of local anesthesia and nitrous oxide. There are over 200 independent practices throughout Canada, with 50% of them located in Ontario (Wright, 2009). In Denmark, Italy, Norway and Sweden, independent practice is the sole method of practice and is available along with other types of supervision in other counties, but not all, throughout the world (Johnson, 2009, 72).

ALTERNATIVE SETTINGS   In many cases, less supervision is needed in public health settings or institutions. For example, dental hygienists in Illinois can treat nursing home residents without the physical presence of a dentist. However, the dentist must have examined the patient and provided written orders within 90 days before the initiation of dental hygiene treatment, and the dental hygienist must review the medical history and perform an exam (Illinois Department of Professional Regulation, 2004). Other states, provinces and countries require the *dentist of record* or the patient's dentist to authorize or prescribe procedures; however, the dentist does not need to by physically present. More information on supervision is discussed in Chapter 9.

Some states allow pit and fissure sealants to be done without supervision; other states require a dentist to be present. A state may require the dentist to be physically present if the sealant is applied in private practice but not in other health care settings or on Native Indian reserves. Or a state may indicate that the sealant can be placed under *general supervision* (e.g., in a school or public health setting) if the dentist has *authorized* the sealant and has seen the patient within a given number of days. Box 5-13 defines the four basic levels of supervision applicable to dental hygiene practice.

BOX 5-13

Levels of Supervision in Dental Hygiene Practice Settings

• General supervision	The dentist authorizes the procedures
	The dentist does not have to be physically present
• Indirect supervision	The dentist authorizes the procedures
	The dentist is physically present
• Direct supervision	The dentist authorizes the procedures
	The dentist is physically present
	The dentist approves the work after completion
• Unsupervised	No supervision by dentist
	No authorization by dentist

RESTRICTIONS   Some states have additional restrictions on practicing without a dentist. For example, in Ohio, a dental hygienist may qualify for approval to work without the dentists being physically present in the private dental office setting. This approval is based on years of experience, a course in the identification and prevention of medical emergencies, certification in CPR, and a statement from a licensed dentist that the dental hygienist is competent to work without supervision. But there are restrictions to this mode of practice. For example, it is allowed for no more than 15 consecutive working days (or 3 consecutive weeks of 5 working days per week). There are also set time limits for examination of patients by dentists before dental hygiene treatment, and the dental hygienist should comply with the dentist's written orders. In addition, it must be documented that the patient was informed that the dentist would not be present during dental hygiene treatment (Ohio State Dental Board, 2000). In these circumstances, the patient would be able to choose between supervised and unsupervised dental hygiene treatment. However, if practicing as an expanded dental hygienist and performing restorative procedures, the dentist must be present.

Similarly, in Canada, there are different levels of supervision, and it must be remembered that self-regulation does not always guarantee a reduction or end of supervision. For example, Quebec, the first jurisdiction to have self-regulation in North America, still has direct supervision. In other provinces, the supervision also varies with restrictions, such as setting the designated time in which specific dental hygiene services can be rendered after examination or authorization by a dentist, the established relationship with a dentist, and the specific procedures that must have a dentist present.

COLLABORATIVE PRACTICE   In addition to advocating for less restrictive supervision, dental hygienists are becoming more involved with collaborative practice situations where they work with a consulting dentist as a cotherapist. In this model, dental hygienists and dentists work as colleagues without general supervision (Darby & Walsh, 2010, p. 1217; Daniel, Harfst, & Wilder, 2008, p. 9; Wilkins, 2009, p. 4). Box 5-14 defines the decision making responsibilities along with the levels of supervision. See Chapter 9 for more discussion on the collaborative practice model.

Both Canada and the United States have recent and ongoing initiatives to reduce the level of supervision. One major reason for this can be attributed to the need to increase access to preventive dental hygiene services in settings and geographic areas where the supervision of a dentist is a

BOX 5-14

Decision-making Responsibilities

- Dentist
  Dentist decides all procedures to be provided
  Dentist can be on-site or off-site
- Collaborative
  Dental hygienist and dentist together decide services
  Dentist can be on-site or off-site
- Independent
  Dental hygienist decides services and refers as necessary
  Dentist is not required

(Johnson, 2009, p.71).

hindrance to individuals receiving care (see Chapter 6). Another reason for less restrictive supervision is to enhance the status of dental hygiene as a profession due to the fact that dental hygienists would not be supervised by another profession, which also is the major employer (Lautar, 1995). Factors affected by legislative or regulatory requirements of supervision are outlined in Box 5-15.

At present, the ADHA is proposing a new level of dental hygienist: the advanced dental hygiene practitioner. This will be a dental hygienist who has taken additional training (the curriculum is presently being developed). This new oral health provider will serve the unmet needs of the public by working in settings that will improve access to oral health care and by providing restorative and preventive procedures, especially for underserved populations, including Medicaid recipients (American Dental Hygienists' Association, 2005). Variations on this mid-level provider are

BOX 5-15

Factors Affecting Levels of Supervision

- The geographic location (state, province, territory, country)
- The setting in which services are delivered (i.e., private-practice dental office, public health center, long-term care facility, prison, school)
- The circumstances under which services are provided (i.e., in the presence or absence of a dentist)
- The kinds of services that can be offered (i.e., screenings, education, local anesthesia, sealant, scaling and root planing)
- The patients to whom services are supplied (i.e., nursing home residents, elementary school-children, underserved populations such as Medicaid recipients)

Source: Adapted from Center for Health Workforce Studies (2004, p. 85).

now in Minnesota and Washington. See Chapter 9 for more information on alternative practice models. Globally, dental hygiene is seeing less restriction on supervision and decision-making responsibilities and more career opportunities including expanded duties such as administering local anesthesia, orthodontic banding, bleaching, placing temporary dressings, and providing restorative procedures. There are plans for master programs in dental hygiene outside of the United States; in Norway there are plans for a doctorate in dental hygiene (Johnson, 2009).

FORENSIC DENTISTRY

Dental forensics and forensic odontology are terms used interchangeably in the field of forensic dentistry (Voelker, 2009, p. 58). **Forensic dentistry** is the dental specialty that uses evidence such as bite marks, human teeth, and dental records to identify human remains, assess injuries, and provide other facts or data in criminal or civil cases. This specialty works with legal cases (i.e., physical abuse) and disaster situations (i.e., fires, terrorism, earthquakes, hurricanes, and accidents). Evidence such as bite marks, saliva DNA, and head, face, and month injuries (documented by radiographs, photographs, descriptions and other dental records) are used. The next chapter, Chapter 6, outlines signs of abuse.

The important roles that good dental records and thorough documentation play cannot be under-estimated. The verification of the smallest amount of dental evidence, especially since tooth structures such as enamel are stronger than other body tissues, has the ability to determine a series of events, guilt or innocence, or the identification of bodily remains. Dental records (i.e., radiographs and charting) are used to compare post-mortem (after death) data with ante-mortem (before death) data. Findings that would be compared include decayed, missing, and filled teeth, along with tooth anatomy such as root morphology (Voekler, 2009, p. 59). Bite marks are used to identify the abuser (who may bite the victim or is bitten by the victim) and any item that might have been bitten by the perpetrator at the crime scene.

Dental hygienists are able to obtain more training in forensic dentistry through continuing education courses and membership in professional organizations such as the American Academy of Forensic Sciences. Dental hygienists are able to participate in the five main areas of forensic dentistry due to their background in gathering and recording information from dental radiographs and clinical dental conditions. The five areas are listed in Box 5-16.

BOX 5-16

Forensic Dentistry Areas

- Personal identification by means of dental records
- Disaster victim identification in mass casualty incidents
- Human bite mark analysis
- Recognition and analysis of the injuries associated with family violence
- Professional negligence and dental standards of care

(Ferguson, Sweet, & Craig, 2008).

Summary

The practice of dental hygiene involves not only the ethical considerations discussed in the previous chapters but also legal considerations. Dental hygienists not practicing in accordance with the dental practice act, which is legislated law, may be liable in criminal court. Dental hygienists may also be liable in civil court if they commit actions against individuals such as malpractice, defamation, technical assault, and breach of contract. With the exception of Alabama, dental hygienists must graduate from an accredited dental hygiene program, pass a written exam, and, depending on the jurisdictions (state or province), pass a practical exam to be licensed. Dental and dental hygiene practice acts outline the rules and regulations for the practice of dental hygiene. Levels of supervision vary according to geographic jurisdictions, procedures or services, treatment settings, and the type of patients. Globally, dental hygienists are advancing the profession. One area where dental hygienists can be used is forensic dentistry.

Critical Thinking

1. Compare two state or two provincial dental/dental hygiene practice acts. What similarities do you find between the two acts regarding the practice of dental hygiene (e.g., continuing education requirements, supervision level, allowable procedures, fee payment, licensing body, and so on)? Report the findings to the class.
2. Debate the issue of levels of supervision found in a practice act. Do you feel that one standard is appropriate for one setting and not for another? Why do you think a dental practice act is written with the various levels of supervision?
3. Name the levels of supervision for a dental hygienist. In your state or province, does the level of supervision change with the procedures performed, the location where the procedures are performed, or the population served?
4. Give an example in which a dental hygienist may be charged with a crime against society under criminal law. Give another example in which a dental hygienist may be charged with a crime against an individual under civil law.
5. What are the conditions necessary to make a contract binding?
6. Define the key terms found at the beginning of this chapter. Apply each term to a situation applicable to the practice of dental hygiene.
7. Taking into account both the ethical and the legal considerations, compare the rights of patients, duties of providers owed to patients, and duties of patients owed to providers, such as dental hygienists.
8. Discuss the emerging areas of dental hygiene, including forensic dentistry.

CHAPTER 6

Social Issues

OBJECTIVES

After reading the material in this chapter, you will be able to

- Identify legislation that protects and aids the patient and the dental hygienist against discrimination in dentistry.
- Recognize the signs of abuse (child, spouse, and elderly).
- List barriers to access to care and reasons for disparities in oral health care.
- Discuss the advantages and disadvantages of various reimbursement or insurance plans (Medicaid, Medicare, and managed care) as they pertain to access to care and distributive justice issues.
- Discuss the role of the dental hygienist as an advocate for oral health care.

KEY TERMS

Access to care

Advocate

Child abuse

Culture

Disparities

Distributive justice

Domestic violence

Elderly abuse

Managed care

Medicaid

Medicare

Sexual harassment

Spouse abuse

INTRODUCTION

Ethical and legal issues often overlap; an issue can be both ethical and legal. Similarly, ethical and legal issues can also be integrated into social issues. Social issues that dental hygienists must sometimes deal with are related to obligations to society and to the problems of the workplace. Among the social issues addressed in this chapter are employment laws, reporting of abuse, and access to care. In addition to laws that govern the practice of dental hygiene and patient treatment that were discussed in Chapter 5, there are federal and state laws that protect individuals in the workplace. Violations of these laws or acts can be judged throughout the various levels of the judicial system. Antidiscrimination laws not only protect dental hygienists in the workplace but also enable patients to receive equal quality of care.

Another social issue that involves both ethical and legal responsibilities is the ability to recognize abuse and the mandate to report such abuse. Access to care is a social issue with legal and ethical ramifications. Barriers to access to care are financial, geographical, and sociological, including cultural barriers. Government documents, laws and mandates make recommendations to decrease the health care disparities found among population groups. The dental hygienist can play a role as an **advocate** in increasing access to oral health care, especially among the underserved populations.

Case Study

You have been working part-time in private dental practice for the past five years since the birth of your first child. Your child is now enrolled in kindergarten and you are a volunteer parent at the school helping regularly on your days off. As you work with children in the various grades, you notice many of them have poor oral hygiene and visible decay. You speak to the school nurse about this. She is aware of the problem but is unable to find dentists in the area who will treat children on Medicaid or the parents are unable to afford their children's dental care.

The community has a diverse population with some households making over $100,000 (being two-income families) and well-educated parents with graduate degrees. Other households are below the poverty line due to unemployment and low-skilled jobs. Fifty percent of the school's population is on *free and reduced-price* lunches. The school is located in a rural area where many of the families live on farmland that has been in the family for years. The teachers are dedicated and many of them were raised in the vicinity, and they have known each other and the parents for many years.

As you read this chapter, consider the following: What are some actions you can take to improve the oral health status of these children with poor oral hygiene and dental decay?

WORKPLACE LEGISLATION

There exists legislation to protect both the patient and the employee. Unfortunately, because of the small number of employees working at private dental offices, some laws do not apply to dental hygienists. Frequently, where a federal law may not apply, a state may protect the sole employee. MyHealthProfessionsKit with this textbook lists sources for more information regarding employment rights. A portion of this chapter will discuss some workplace laws that pertain to dental hygiene practice. There are many other legal regulations that are applicable to dental hygienists, including minimum wage, unemployment and retirement benefits, taxes, and employment contracts. These will be discussed in Chapters 10 and 11.

Affirmative Action

According to Title VII of the Civil Rights Act of 1964, an individual cannot be discriminated against because of race, color, religion, national origin, gender, or pregnancy. This act applies to the treatment of patients; that is, a health care provider cannot refuse treating a patient on the basis of these criteria. This act also protects the dental hygienist as an employee. If a dental hygienist feels that he or she is discriminated against, the individual should contact the Equal Employment Opportunity Commission. Examples of discrimination include unfair denial of a job, denial of a deserved promotion, or not getting equal pay.

Dental hygienists may be especially vulnerable to discrimination in the private dental practice setting because they often rely on one person for employment: the dentist. In private offices that employ few workers, there are no strict regulations for hiring, promoting, or rewarding employees as there are for large organizations. The dentist ultimately decides who gets hired, the working conditions, and salary. Dental hygienists in private practice may find themselves in a difficult situation where one person has the authority of making all decisions that affect their careers. For example, two dental hygienists working in the same office and doing equal work in terms of patient treatment may not be paid the same salary. Although there is a moral obligation for the dentist to do so, there is no legal process to ensure equal pay, particularly in practices that employ only a few dental hygienists. It may also happen that one dental hygienist has more experience or more education: in that case, should he or she be paid more? Again, what one dentist does another may not, and there are no rigid rules to be followed.

Other situations may also raise questions about discrimination in the private office. For example, what happens if the male dental hygienist in the office does equal work but receives a higher salary? Or, as a dental hygienist gets older, would it be justified to replace him or her with a younger person? There are no strict guidelines to address such practices, but the dental hygienist who is treated unfairly may sue. The problem is that in employment settings involving a small number of workers, affirmative action is not always applicable. However, this does not mean that dental hygienists are totally powerless. They can appeal to courts of law for correcting discriminatory practices.

Pregnancy Discrimination Act

Dental hygienists are especially vulnerable to pregnancy discrimination; dental hygiene is a female-dominated profession with 99% of practicing dental hygienists being women (ADHA, 2009). A woman cannot be fired or denied a job because of pregnancy, childbirth, or related medical conditions, according to the Pregnancy Discrimination Act of 1978. If her pregnancy limits her job function, she must be granted the same job considerations as others with similar limitations or abilities. While on pregnancy leave, a pregnant employee must receive the same benefits given to other employees on leaves (e.g., vacation, pay increases, and seniority). This act is very important for dental hygienists because it prohibits an employer from forcing a pregnant dental hygienist to take maternity leave either before or after birth. It also imposes an obligation on the employer to hold the job open for the same length of time as for other employees on sick or disability leave. A dentist could replace the dental hygienist while she is on maternity leave, and that is not against the law as long as it is a temporary replacement. But the law forbids permanent replacement of a pregnant employee.

Family and Medical Leave Act

This federal act, referred to as FMLA, allows leaves of absence of up to twelve unpaid weeks of salary for the employee after using all vacation pay and sick leave. Leave of absence is applicable for birth or adoption, serious illness, or care of a family member. Dental hygienists, the majority of whom are women, often have family responsibilities, commitments, and obligations that are protected by this act. Women are the ones who are usually expected to care for children as well as for sick family members. This law covers full-time workers in workplaces with fifty or more employees. Thus, family medical leaves may not be applicable to the majority of dental hygienists. In fact, only those who work for organizations (e.g., companies, hospitals, government agencies, public health departments, and educational institutions) can benefit from this law.

Americans with Disabilities Act

There are two sides to disability. First, disabled patients should not be discriminated against. Second, disabled dental hygienists should be protected from discrimination in the workplace. A *disability* is a condition that interferes with life functions. In dental hygiene practice, care providers cannot withhold treatment or provide less quality of treatment to a disabled patient. This would be discrimination. However, we must recognize the difference between treating a patient with a disability and treating a medically compromised patient who may need to be treated in special facilities or by specialists. At times, there is a need to use different procedures for disabled patients in order to provide quality of care and standard of care. For example, a patient with AIDS can be treated safely in a dental practice because of the effectiveness of standard precautions, while a patient with hemophilia may need to be treated in a hospital if the procedure is invasive because of the risk of bleeding. It is an ethical duty to treat those in need of care, but at the same time one should not risk harm to a patient with a special condition, to other patients, or to oneself.

DISABLED PATIENTS   The question at this point is, Is the treatment provided to a disabled (or special needs) patient the same as to the nondisabled patients? For example, if the dental hygienist does not double-glove for all patients, then he or she should not double-glove for a medically compromised patient or a patient with a communicable disease. If standard precautions (replaces the term universal precautions) are used, there is no need to base infection control on known or perceived infectious status of the patient (Daniel, Harfst & Wilder, 2008, p. 892). Although gloving does provide a barrier against infections, some providers prefer to double-glove to decrease operator exposure and inner-glove perforation during high-risk oral surgeries (Schwimmer, Massoumi, & Barr, 1994). To double-glove based on the individual patient and not the procedure would be discriminatory. However, if the dental hygienist feels that the patient's health status would be compromised or does not have the skills, equipment, or experience to treat a medically compromised patient and has consulted with the patient's physician, then referral could be justified (Weinstein, 1993, p. 84). Health care providers not only must treat the disabled, they also must provide accessibility. Dental offices should be accessible through wheelchair ramps and elevators. The more recently constructed or renovated operatories accommodate wheelchairs.

DISABLED EMPLOYEES   Now it is appropriate to examine the other side of the issue of disability, that is, how the Americans with Disabilities Act applies to dental hygienists in the workplace. The rights of people with disabilities were protected by the Rehabilitation Act of 1973. At first, this act applied only to employers or institutions that contracted with the federal government or received federal funding. Only the handicapped employees of these employers were covered by the act. Later, bloodborne infectious diseases became recognized as handicaps. In 1990, the Americans with Disabilities Act applied the same standards as the Rehabilitation Act and extended it to private employers not receiving federal funding.

As small businesses, dental offices do not have to comply with all the provisions of the Americans with Disabilities Act in terms of hiring. However, a dental hygienist cannot be disqualified from a position based on a disability, such as being confined to a wheelchair, as long as the dental hygienist can perform the ordinary (usual) duties. According to this act, it is the responsibility of the employer or business (e.g., the private-practice dentist) to make structural changes to the office or purchase any special equipment required for the disabled person to perform the job (Ganssle, 1995, p. 24). Judgments have been made concerning dental hygienists who are medically compromised that may have an effect on their patients. In the case of a dental hygienist being infected with HIV (a fatal, contagious disease) and working with and sharp instruments are in the patient's mouth, it was determined that HIV does present a threat to the workplace and the dental hygienist is not qualified under Americas with Disabilities Act (Palmer, 2002, p. 27).

EQUIPMENT ADJUSTMENTS   In interviews with paraplegic dental hygienists, Seckman (2000) found that the foot-operated rheostat of the dental hand piece presents a major problem for them. However, dental equipment manufacturers are receptive to the idea of altering equipment for the disabled. In addition, asepsis (e.g., regloving) does not seem to be a problem if dental hygienists use electric wheelchairs and cover the joystick with a bag. Needed equipment can be obtained through various agencies, such as state departments of vocational rehabilitation. A support group or network of dental hygienists practicing in wheelchairs has been suggested to help the newly injured provider continue practicing dental hygiene (Zimmermann, 2002). If a dental hygienist or any other potential employee feels discriminated against, an attorney should be consulted.

Age Discrimination in Employment Act

The Age Discrimination in Employment Act prohibits employment discrimination based on age in businesses employing twenty or more workers, so this act protects dental hygienists over forty years of age only in large facilities. The problem is that the dental office usually does not have twenty or more employees and therefore is not included under this act. However, the Age Discrimination Act of 1975, a national law, prohibits discrimination on the basis of age in programs or activities receiving federal financial assistance, such as health care and human service providers. This law may cover more dental hygienists as they become employed in the nontraditional dental hygiene practice settings that receive federal funding.

Sexual Harassment

Any unwelcome or unwanted behavior or activities of a sexual nature that occur between two or more individuals of unequal power is considered **sexual harassment**. Because males usually have higher positions of power in the workforce, sexual harassment is considered a form of sex discrimination. Therefore, sexual harassment is a violation of the Civil Rights Act.

In a study of Washington dental hygienists, over 25% of the respondents had experienced harassment by either dentists or patients, and 35% knew of other oral health care staff who had been harassed. In addition, 23% of those harassed terminated employment by resigning or quitting rather than by being fired (Garvin & Siedge, 1992, p. 183). Years later, when Virginia dental hygienists were surveyed, over half of the responding dental hygienists indicated that they had experienced sexual harassment. Although 70% of the respondents perceived filing a formal complaint as strategy for managing sexual harassment, less than 1% of these dental hygienists did so (Pennington, Darby, Bauman, Plichta, & Schnuth, 2000, p. 288). In a survey of graduating senior dental hygiene students, 86% felt it their responsibility to report it if they observed it in the dental office; however, 92% would report sexual harassment if directed at them (Duley et al. 2009, p. 351).

Sexual harassment in the dental office may be between a male dentist who has power as the employer and a female dental hygienist who is a subordinate employee; the harassment may also come from a patient or colleague of the opposite sex. It can be between a female dentist and a male dental hygienist or between two individuals of the same sex, as well as between a dental hygienist and a patient. There can also be informal sexual harassment, where there is no formal hierarchy of power, such as between two students or two coworkers of equal status. It is important to note that sexual harassment tends to be a repeated behavior. For example, a one-time comment made in a joke may not be considered harassment, but repeated unwelcomed comments of a sexual nature constitute harassment. The one-time joke may also be considered harassment if it makes another individual uncomfortable even as a first-time occurrence.

REPORTING SEXUAL HARASSMENT   Documenting sexual harassment is very important and should include the nature and description of the offensive behaviors and the dates, times, and names. In addition, it is important to inform the offending individual (the person doing the harassing) that the behavior is unwelcome and to tell the immediate supervisor of the incidents. In the dental office, the dentist is the supervisor, so if the dentist is the one doing the harassing, the dental hygienist should inform a partner or an associate in the dental office or the office manager (McKee, 2000; Knight, 2010). If another employee is harassing an individual while functioning under the terms of employment and the supervisor does nothing about it, the supervisor may be also held accountable or liable for the harassment through *respondeat superior* (see definition in Chapter 5).

ADDITIONAL EXAMPLES   The workplace is not the only environment where sexual harassment can occur and is not tolerated by law. For example, the Illinois Human Rights Act protects employees and higher education students from sexual harassment. Furthermore, public contractors and bidders are required to have a written policy about sexual harassment. And, even if one is trying to settle the claim of sexual harassment through the union or some other internal grievance, a charge still must be claimed with the Department of Human Rights (Illinois Department of Human Rights, 2010).

Occupational Safety and Health Act

The Occupational Safety and Health Admistration (OSHA) is a result of the Occupational Safety and Health Act of 1970. The purpose of this act is to ensure a safe and healthy workplace, while "OSHA is responsible for administering the Act, issuing standards, and conducting on-site inspections to ensure compliance with the Act" (Pozgar, 2004, p. 439). Even before you started dental hygiene education (and probably as a requirement for dental hygiene clinic courses), you followed procedures outlined in the bloodborne standard. For example, your dental hygiene program may have asked for proof of a hepatitis B vaccine. Later in your dental hygiene studies, you received training in standard precautions, bloodborne pathogens, and OSHA guidelines. These and other measures are enforced in order to follow protocols set by OSHA. The guidelines may remain the same or may change as you continue in dental hygiene or switch careers. For example, the Bloodborne Pathogen Standard of 1991 was revised in response to the Needlestick Safety and Prevention Act in 2001 (U.S. Department of Labor, 2005).

TRAINING AND INSPECTION   By law, dental hygienists are required to receive initial and annual updated training in bloodborne pathogens, provided at the expense of employers and during working hours. Because private dental offices often have fewer than eleven employees, these workplaces are not routinely inspected. But if OSHA guidelines are not followed in a dental office, regardless of the number of employees, a complaint can be filed, and the dental office will be investigated.

ERGONOMICS   An important aspect of occupational safety for dental hygienists is the role of ergonomics. Dental hygienists are prone to develop carpal tunnel syndrome as a result of the repetitive nature of dental hygiene procedures. This syndrome affects people who perform repetitive movements with their hands. Other musculoskeletal disorders may be preventable or lessened with good positioning and by following OSHA ergonomic standards that directly relate to the specific job activities of the dental hygienist (Daniel, Harfst, & Wilder, 2008, p. 151).

WORKPLACE VIOLENCE   Part of occupational health and safety in the workplace is protection against workplace violence. According to the National Institute for Occupational Safety and Health, homicide is the leading cause of workplace death among females (mainly in convenience stores and as taxi drivers). The most common reasons are robbery and disgruntled spouses. Dental hygienists are at some risk for violence in the workplace, as dental offices have money and drugs. It has been reported that health care facilities are a primary target of violence, especially by drug seekers. According to the U.S. Department of Labor and Industries, there were 8.3 per 10,000 assaults to health care workers as compared to 2 assaults per 10,000 for all private sector industries. McPhaul and Lipscomb (2004) report that the majority of the threats and assaults come from patients or their families and visitors.

The best way for dental hygienists to protect themselves and others against workplace violence is to use common sense. For example, if the office has a back door, it should be kept locked. Dental hygienists should also be aware of patients who are not happy with the services or treatment they have received because they may translate their frustration into violence. As dental hygienists move outside the traditional private-practice settings and into alternative settings, they should be aware of situations that are high risks for workforce violence in various institutional and community settings, such as nursing homes, long-term care facilities, home health, social services, and hospital evironments (Centers for Disease Control, 1997; McPhaul & Lipscomb, 2004).

Recently, there has been an increase in shootings at schools, churches, stores, restaurants, and other places of business or work. An active shooter does not intend to harm one individual, but many in a random or systematic way. There is no other crime involved such as hostage taking or robbery (Johnson, 2006). If an active shooter is on the premises and it is impossible to leave the premise, the best protection is to lock yourself in a room, barricade the door, hide behind or under furniture so that you are not seen through a window, be quiet, and set your cell phone to vibrate (you do not want it to ring, but you want to receive a message or relay a message).

Reporting Domestic Violence

Domestic violence is family violence, or that which occurs in the home or within the family. Domestic violence may also be referred to as family abuse and neglect. Using this broad definition, the three types of domestic violence are:

- child abuse
- spouse/partner abuse
- elderly (or elder) abuse

BOX 6-1

Some Common Signs of Abuse

- Physical
  Unexplained bruises
  Bite marks
  Injuries to head and face

- Emotional
  Withdrawn
  Lack of eye contact with
    abuser

- Neglect
  Dressed improperly
  Lack of personal hygiene
  Denied medical/dental care

Abuse can also occur outside the home, such as in day care facilities and nursing homes. At times, the term *domestic violence* is reserved for spouse abuse. It is the dental hygienist's ethical and legal responsibility to recognize the signs of abuse and to report cases of abuse to the authorities in accordance with the regulations. In many states, dental hygienists are mandated reporters of abuse. In a survey of graduating dental hygienists, 94% of the respondents agreed or strongly agreed that it was their responsibility to report observed or suspected child or elder abuse or neglect. However, 85% of the respondents agreed or strongly agreed that it was their responsibility to report spouse or partner abuse (Duley, Fitzpatrick, Zornosa, Lambert, & Mitchell, 2009, p. 349).

Signs of abuse (see Box 6-1) also need to be documented to help the forensic odontologist with identification of the abuser and to be reported to Child Protection Services or law enforcement (Wilkins, 2009, p. 955; Darby, & Walsh, 2010, p. 1140).

Child Abuse

Child abuse is any act that endangers or impairs a child's physical or emotional health or development. In most states, dental hygienists, like other health care professionals, are mandated by law to report child abuse to government authorities. Many states in fact require continuing education on the subject of child abuse. Dental hygienists should know the law and protocol for reporting child abuse. Even in cases of suspected child abuse, providers are given immunity from liability (cannot be sued for falsely reporting in good faith); they can be prosecuted for *not* reporting child abuse (Saxe & McCourt, 1991). In addition, dental hygienists are ethically responsible for protecting these children under the principle of *beneficence* to benefit the patient. Coalitions such as Prevent Abuse and Neglect through Dental Awareness have been instituted to increase awareness and education among dental health care providers, including dental hygienists.

SIGNS   Warning signs of child abuse are repeated injuries (multiple bruises); unusual sites for accidental bumps and bruises; inappropriate behavior by the child; neglected appearance; strict, unduly critical parents; and extremely isolated families. Sixty-five percent of all child abuse injuries include trauma to the head, neck, or mouth (American Dental Association, 1998, p. 33). Therefore, dental hygienists and other dental health care providers are able to detect signs of child abuse. Indications of child abuse that are located outside the mouth include bruises, belt marks, cigarette burns, and bite marks.

The most frequent oral injuries are fractured teeth, laceration of the lingual and labial frenula (frenum) due to forced feeding, missing teeth for which there is no obvious explanation, displaced teeth, discolored teeth, and abnormalities of appearance and mobility of the tongue. Other damage to the tongue, fractures of the maxillary and mandible, and bruised or scarred abrasions at the corners of the mouth are also common (Fonseca & Idelberg, 1993, p. 136; Saxe & McCourt, 1991, p. 363). Signs of sexual abuse may also be found in the mouth, such as erythema and spetechiae of the palate as well as lesions of sexually transmitted diseases. When in doubt about the nature of lesions, a dental hygienist should seek consultation to avoid false accusations.

NEGLECT   Signs of neglect, such as dressing a child for the wrong type of weather or lack of personal hygiene, may also be apparent. Child abuse can also include dental neglect, which is the willful failure of a parent or guardian to seek and follow through with treatment necessary to ensure a level of oral health essential for adequate function and freedom from pain and infections. This type of child abuse can be reported in the same manner as physical abuse. Caution should be used to avoid confusing signs of neglect with the inability to afford the cost of care or other barriers to access to care that are beyond the parent's control. Likewise, religious beliefs may also be responsible for neglect. In the case where a child's life is endangered, the state, through court order, may order the care or treatment to prevent or remedy serious harm to the child. This may also include treatment so that the child is likely to enjoy a higher quality or more normal life (Oral, 2004).

DOCUMENTING   Documentation of abuse is important. In addition to recording in the child's chart a description of the injury (i.e., size, shape, location, and color), a photograph and radiographs may also be taken, although these require the permission of a parent or guardian. If taking a photograph is not possible, sketch the sign of abuse. In cases of suspected child abuse, parental permission may not be needed to take photographs and X-rays in some states. Dental hygienists should know what is legally allowed without parental permission according to the relevant state laws (e.g., health and safety codes, health practice acts, penal codes, and child abuse reporting acts).

INFORMATION GATHERING   The practitioner should ask the child what happened (if possible, without the parent's presence) and then ask the parent what happened. This should be done in a nonthreatening and nonaccusatory way, as the parent may not be aware of the abuse if it is from another caretaker. A threatening confrontation could also spark an angry reaction from the parent. However, hesitation or hostile answers from the parent, conflicting stories from the child and parent, or inconsistency between the parent's account and the injury may be cause for suspicion. For example, an injury that is claimed to have happened yesterday would not be yellow in color; multi-color bruises should raise the index of suspicion. The parent's and child's stories should also be documented. The dental health care provider may also consult with other health professionals, such as the family physician or other primary care provider.

REPORTING   After reporting the incident to the proper authorities (e.g., state child protection agency or child abuse hotline) by phone, the dental health care provider may need to send the necessary documentation. It is important to be familiar with the reporting regulations in the state where one practices dental hygiene. Although it is the mandate of social services to investigate reported cases, the dental health care provider should follow up on the reported case of child abuse. The dental hygienist may discuss suspicions and precautions with the supervising or employing dentist before reporting child abuse.

Some feel that reporting child abuse should be done when there is certainty, as it can be easily mistaken and its reporting can cause much distress and upheaval to the family. Others feel that any suspicion should be taken seriously. Dealing with individual cases requires using the prudent judgment of the dental hygienist. It is important to remember that even if the supervising dentist or other office personnel do not want to get involved, the dental hygienist has both a legal and a moral duty to report child abuse.

Case Study Follow-up #1

In this chapter's cases study, how would you determine which children have neglected dental care that could be classified as child abuse?

Spouse Abuse

The term *domestic violence* covers spouse abuse, battering, or control over an intimate person. **Spouse abuse** (intimate partner violence) is another form of domestic (same-household) violence. It happens to women (as victims) more often than to men. Abuse of women can include either spouse or partner abuse or dating violence (Wilkins, 2009, p. 953). As in the case of child abuse, there are laws in some states that require health care providers to report spouse abuse. However, reporting these incidents is more problematic than reporting incidents of child abuse because the suspected victim can sue for breach of confidentiality if he or she was not consulted first. The suspected victim may claim that the report was filed against his or her will. In this case, there is no liability protection for the dental hygienist (American Dental Association, 1998, p. 23). Therefore, spouse abuse should not be reported without the consent of the abused spouse.

ABUSIVE BEHAVIOR The majority of spouse abuse occurs to the female (battered woman). She may be abused by someone with whom she has been intimate, such as a husband or a significant other. The abuse usually starts with controlling behavior from the abusive spouse; this behavior escalates and becomes more frequent and more aggressive. The dental hygienist should attempt to question the suspected abused patient away from the partner, document findings, speak to the patient in a nonjudgmental way, and have another staff corroborate any suspected findings. In a survey of indiviudals staying at a domestic violencs shelter, 86.6% reported that they were not aksed about their injuries although signs of abuse were present; only 13.3% were asked about their injuries (Nelms, Gutman, Solomon, DeWald, & Campbell, 2009, p. 493). Box 6-2 gives examples of questions to ask the patient that the dental hygienist may use in either a direct or an indirect way. The dental hygienist needs to be supportive when asking these questions and to act as a resource for the abused patient.

DOCUMENTING Among the signs of spouse abuse that can be identified by the dental hygienist are injuries involving the face, eyes, and neck. These may be detected during routine dental hygiene care. The health care provider should be suspicious of repeated bruises, broken bones, cigarette burns, human bite marks, and other signs similar to those found in child abuse. Again, it is very important to document cases of suspected spouse abuse.

REPORTING However, unlike child abuse, not all states have laws that mandate health care providers to report spouse abuse. But ethically, dental hygienists are required, through the principle of beneficence, to *benefit* the patient and promote his or her well-being. So if reporting spouse abuse in a state is not mandated, the dental hygienist should offer advice and support.

BOX 6-2

SAFE Questions

Using the SAFE acronym, these questions are easily remembered:

> *S = Stress/Safety:* Does the patient feel safe? Stressed? Is there a concern for safety?
>
> *A = Afraid/Abused:* Does the patient feel afraid? Has the patient or child been abused or threatened?
>
> *F = Friends/Family:* Do the family and friends of the patient know about the abuse? Will they give the patient support? How isolated is the patient?
>
> *E = Emergency Plan:* Does the patient have an emergency plan? Would the patient like to have one? Does the patient know where a shelter is located? Does the patient have a safe place and resources for an emergency?

(Ashur, 1993, p. 2367; Gibson-Howell, 1996, p. 79).

COWORKERS   In addition to patients, coworkers can also be at risk for spouse abuse, especially as the majority of employees in dental offices are women. Training sessions in the recognition of domestic violence, documentation, and referral should be addressed in the workplace. Likewise, an environment of support, trust, and confidentiality should be maintained.

Elderly Abuse

Another form of abuse is **elderly abuse** (sometimes referred to as elder abuse). This occurs when a relative (i.e., child, spouse, or other family member) or a health care provider abuses a geriatric patient. Elderly abuse can be physical, sexual, emotional, confinement, passive neglect, willful deprivation, and financial exploitation. The most common form of elderly abuse is financial, which includes taking money, using the elderly person's property or possessions without permission, and scams such as telemarketing (Herrren & Bryon, 2005). For example, a child, the primary care provider, or another person may cash the social security check of an elderly person and spend it for personal use rather than for the needs of the elderly individual.

SIGNS   More than half of the abusers are the primary caregivers (Elderly Abuse and Neglect Program, 1991) such as an adult child. As with child and spouse abuse, dental hygienists should look for signs of physical abuse. These could include unexplained or unusual injuries, lack of appropriate dress or personal hygiene, and behavior that reflects abuse, such as being withdrawn or suspicious of the dental hygienist as a result of losing trust in others. In addition, the behavior of a caretaker who accompanies an elderly patient may raise suspicion, such as not allowing an older individual to speak for himself or herself. Fearful or intimidated behavior on the part of the abused should also raise suspicion (see Box 6-1) as well as change in behavior. For example, a patient who was previously upbeat is now sad and uncommunicative (Turchetta, 2008, p. 48).

REPORTING   Suspected elderly abuse should be reported to the local social service agency that deals with aging or elderly abuse and neglect. In some states, dental hygienists are mandated to report elderly abuse in the same way they are suppose to report child abuse. It is necessary to document findings similarly to child abuse and spouse abuse. As the elderly population grows and relies on health care providers, it is important that the dental hygienist be aware of potential elderly abuse, its signs, and how to confront the situation legally and ethically. Unfortunately, as Murphree et al. (2002) found, most dental hygienists are not prepared to recognize and report elderly abuse. In this study, only 20.5% of the responding dental hygienists scored a 78% or higher on a nine-item fact quiz with the average grade of 46.2% (p. 1277).

One of the problems associated with reporting elderly abuse is that the elderly person may not want the dental hygienist to report the abuse. This can be a difficult situation. For example, if the abuser is a child of the abused, the elderly individual may not want to report the actions of a son or daughter. In addition, elderly persons may think of the consequences of reporting abuse and worry about losing any type of positive relationship they have with those who take care of them. Or the victim may be financially dependent upon the abuser, which is a common factor in elder abuse (Turchetta, 2008, p. 48).

Many states have legislation that facilitates the reporting of elderly abuse. For example, the Illinois Elderly Abuse and Neglect Act protects reporters and caseworkers from civil or criminal liability (Illinois Department on Aging, 1999). There are many local agencies available for support and information. In most situations, the local social service agencies can help the abused. If one cannot find a local agency that can help an elderly abused patient, the individual should contact the American Association of Retired Persons, a national advocate organization for senior citizens (www.aarp.org).

ACCESS TO CARE

Although the United States may be viewed as a country with good health care in terms of medical technology and skilled practitioners, Americans lack easy, affordable **access to care**. It is estimated that the uninsured rate of Americans is approximately 15% (Turner, Boudreaux, & Lynch, 2009, p. 8). Access to care is an individual's ability to obtain timely personal health services to achieve the best possible health outcomes (Public Health Futures Illinois, 2000, p. 89). Other developed countries are able to provide more health services to more people and to have a healthier population at less cost (Shi & Singh, 2010, p. 11). The problems with access to care apply also to oral health. It has been only in recent years that awareness of the dental needs of the American population has surfaced at the national level. Examples of documents that outline access to care issues are found in Box 6-3.

Disparities

Disparities exist when there are inequalities between groups, such as a difference in health or in health care due to socioeconomic conditions, age, race, and so on. For example, minority children are less likely than U.S. born children, and children who live in rural areas are less likely than urban children, to have dental insurance (Liu, Probst, Wang, & Salinas, 2007). Federal governments have attempted to improve the health care of their citizens. *Healthy People 2010: Objectives for Impoving Health* (U.S. Department of Health and Human Services, 2000a) outlined goals to achieve a healthy population, including one for oral health: to prevent and control oral and craniofacial diseases, conditions, and injuries and improve access to related services, including seventeen objectives. An updated *Healthy People 2020* is currently being drafted, and many of the same goals will remain.

BOX 6-3

Examples

- Current studies have indicated that oral health is an indicator of overall health; research has shown correlation of periodontal disease with other health problems, such as heart disease and low-term birth rates (Loesche, 1997). Consequently, the status of dental health within a population is an indicator of the status of general health in that population.
- *Oral Health in America: A Report of the Surgeon General*, released on May 25, 2000, included for the first time a report on oral health (U.S. Department of Health and Human Services, 2000b).
- The Canadian Dental Hygienists Association also has a position paper on the link between oral health and general health titled "Your Mouth: Portal to Your Body" (Lux & Lavigne, 2004). This paper can be viewed at *http://www.cdha.ca.*
- Both the American Dental Hygienists' Association and the Canadian Dental Hygienists Association have "Access to Care" position papers available on their Web sites.

INTERNATIONAL DISPARITIES   Canadians have made recommendations for their health care system in the document *Building on Values: The Future of Health Care in Canada* (Health Canada, 2002). Both of these documents speak to access-to-care issues and disparities among population groups, including women, the elderly, rural residents, minorities, the disabled, and other diverse population groups. Internationally, the World Health Organization has also published a report that "outlines [the] current oral health situation at a global level and the strategies and approaches for better oral health in the 21st centrury" (World Health Organization, 2003).

Responding to the U.S. Surgeon General's Report on Oral Health, a framework titled *A National Call to Action to Promote Oral Health* (U.S. Department of Health and Human Services, 2003) was introduced to reduce health disparities, promote health and prevent disease, and improve quality of life. Five specific actions recommended in this document are outlined in Box 6-4.

BOX 6-4

Recommendations to Decrease Disparities

- Change perceptions of oral health
- Overcome barriers by replicating effective programs and proven efforts
- Build the science base and accelerate science transfer
- Increase oral health workforce diversity, capacity, and flexibility
- Increase collaborations

Source: A National Call to Action, U.S. Department of Health and Human Services (2003).

Financial Barriers

One of the ten leading health indicators named in *Healthy People 2010* is access to health care. One of the major barriers to access to care is the lack of financial resources. The uninsured cannot afford to be sick or to seek preventive services. It is alarming that the number of those without dental insurance is three times the number of those without health insurance. That is, access to dental care is much more limited than access to general health care. It is speculated that a universal health care system may solve the financial problem; however, it may not solve all the access problems, such as transportation, distance, lack of providers, and an individual's perceived need for treatment. Further measures need to be undertaken to facilitate access to oral health care. To enhance such access, strategies need to be developed that provide dental insurance as well as the means to obtain care.

INSURANCE   Traditionally, dental services, including those of dental hygiene, were reimbursed through fee-for-service. The patient paid the dentist for the treatment received. Later, private dental insurance became available. In this financial arrangement, an individual would pay a premium to the insurance company, which would pay a portion of selected treatment costs, and the patient would pay the balance (called a copayment) and would also be responsible for the cost of procedures not covered by the insurance plan.

Although insurance may help relieve the financial barrier, the worry is that insurance dictates treatment. Based on the restrictions on reimbursement by insurance companies, a dentist may decide to use one type of restorative material or procedure that is less expensive than another regardless of the long-term benefit to the patient. In addition, patients may decide to visit dental hygienists once a year instead of twice or three times because the insurance will pay for only one visit each year. Similarly, if fluoride is not covered under the insurance plan, a parent may not give consent for a child to receive it. Additionally, patients with dental insurance may not seek dental care due to dental anxiety (Sohn & Ismail, 2005).

Insurance can also influence a wide range of policies in the dental office, from who gets a toothbrush to the length of an appointment. It may also affect referrals to a specialist, and some dental insurance plans restrict the care provided by specialists to the most complicated conditions. This is true not only for the dental but also for the medical profession, where the physician or primary care provider is pressured to act as the *gatekeeper* for the insurance company and limits referrals to specialists. Thus, reducing financial barriers through insurance is not without its disadvantages. Box 6-5 gives examples of access-to-care barriers.

BOX 6-5

Examples of Access-to-Care Barriers

- Financial
  Money
  Insurance restrictions

- Location
  Travel restrictions
  Provider availability

- Sociological
  Perceived need
  Language and nonverbal
    communication

BOX 6-6

Managed Care Plans for Dentistry

- Capitation
- Dental health maintenance organization (DHMO)
- Preferred provider organization (PPO)

(Bergmann, 2000, p. 48).

Managed Care

Health maintenance organizations (HMO) are based on the strategy of lowering the cost of care by preventing disease and maintaining health. The idea behind managed care is to get individuals in good health and then to *maintain* that health so that the cost of treatment becomes more affordable. **Managed care** has evolved into a system of health care delivery that controls the utilization and costs of services and that measures performance to deliver quality, cost-effective health care (Public Health Futures Illinois, 2000, p. 93). Managed care plans allow for greater access to care in terms of financial coverage for the patient, although managed care may limit the choice of providers. The three types of managed care plans for dentistry are listed in Box 6-6 and further discussed in Chapter 8.

CAPITATION   One form of managed care is capitation. In this financial system, the dentist contracts with the insurance company to provide services to a given number of individuals enrolled in the managed care plan. The dentist receives a monthly payment based on the number of individuals. The advantage of capitation for the dentist is that it provides a guaranteed income over the entire year. Its advantage for patients is lower cost.

Two problems are associated with this plan. First, the patients are assigned to a certain dentist; thus, a patient has a limited choice in selecting a dentist or is forced to receive care from only that dentist. Second, the dentist receives a set amount of money per patient; thus, the dentist may be forced to use a lower standard of care in terms of cost for treatment procedures or to absorb the cost and lose money. For example, if a patient presents with a need for replacing several amalgam restorations, the dentist has to decide to use amalgam again or to use a higher-cost aesthetic material; obviously, financial factors will influence the decision.

DHMO AND PPO   Another form of a managed care plan is a DHMO. In this plan, a dentist provides all the services specified in the plan to the individuals enrolled in the plan. In the third type of managed care, preferred provider organization (PPO), the patient selects a dentist from a given list of providers. The difference between these two plans and capitation is that, in the former, the dentist is paid for procedures and not according to how many individuals are enrolled in the plan.

Although the American Dental Association is against managed care because it may control treatment of the patient and/or income of the dentist, the American Dental Hygienists' Association is in favor of managed care. Managed care could provide careers for dental hygienists. Those who practice in traditional private dental offices may prefer to move to managed care centers. In addition, more nontraditional roles could be created, such as quality assurance and management utilization review. Moreover, dental hygienists are the preventive experts. If managed care organizations would pay a dental hygienist directly for the services rendered rather than paying through a dentist, money could be saved for the insurance companies while perhaps providing more salary for the dental hygienist. The savings could be used to provide more preventive care to more individuals and to finance more restorative and other types of dental treatments.

Government Assistance

MEDICAID   Government assistance or insurance, known as **Medicaid,** covers indigent or low-income individuals and disabled individuals. Depending upon the state benefits, it may not cover preventive dental services for adults, which would include dental hygiene services. Each state determines how much it will reimburse the dentist for treatment, and this may be limited to emergency procedures or dentures. Under Medicaid, dental services are considered optional services. However, dental screenings are part of the Early and Periodic Screening Diagnosis and Treatment covered by Medicaid for children.

Dentists can elect to participate in Medicaid, but this is optional. An individual may be covered by Medicaid for dental services without being able to obtain the needed dental treatment because the dentist does not accept Medicaid (Nathe, 2005, p. 66). It has been reported that only 20% of the Medicaid-eligible children actually receive preventive oral health services (Peck, 2000, p. 43). The reasons cited by the dental community for not accepting these patients are the low reimbursement by the government and the cumbersome paperwork involved (LeBlanc et al., 1997). Some dentists also state that frequent cancellation of appointments and no-shows by this segment of the population are other reasons for not accepting Medicaid patients. Recently, dental hygienists in some states have become eligible as Medicaid providers and have been able to make an impact both in the number of dental hygiene services rendered and in the number of Medicaid patients seen (American Dental Hygienists' Association, 2004).

SCHIP   In an effort to reach children who may not have private insurance or the financial resources to pay for treatment, the government has instituted the Children's Health Insurance Program or State Children's Health Insurance Program. Each state has its own program under this plan. For example, in Illinois the program is Kid Care. The amount of the insurance premium is based on a sliding scale that considers the number of dependents and annual income of the family. This plan covers not only children but also pregnant women. This is an attempt by the government to provide health care for the uninsured working poor. However, as reported by the *National Survey of Children's Health* nearly one fourth (22.1%) of U.S. children lack dental insurance coverage, over twenty-five percent (26.9%) do have routine preventive care, and five percent (5.1%) have unmet dental needs as indicated by their parents (Liu, Probst, Martin, & Salinas, 2007, p. S12).

MEDICARE   Another form of government assistance or insurance is **Medicare**, the largest health insurance program in the United States. It provides insurance coverage for individuals who are sixty-five years or older, those who are disabled, or those who have permanent organ (i.e., kidney) failure. Medicare provides both hospital and medical insurance. There is limited dental coverage with Medicare; it does not cover routine dental services. However, it does cover certain dental services such as those involved with a fractured jaw, surgical interventions, and cancer radiation therapy (ADA, 2010; Patton, White, & Field, 2001). With an aging population and the high cost of prescription drugs, extending Medicare benefits has generated social and political issues. As a result, the Medicare and Prescription Drug, Improvement, and Modernization Act of 2003 provided drug discount cards starting in May 2004, blood tests for early detection of heart disease and diabetes screening tests since 2005, and provide a prescription drug plan in 2006 (Senior Health, 2004). Medicare benefits have also been expanded to include cost of clinical trails for cancer patients (National Cancer Institute, 2010) and to bridge prescription coverage through the Patient Protection and Affordable Care Act.

The term "Medicare" in Canada is quite different. It is the insurance system in Canada covered by the Canada Health Act; however, it does not cover basic oral health care services (Richardson, 2005).

HEALTH REFORM   In March 2010, the *Patient Protection and Affordable Care Act* was passed in the United States. This act provided medical insurance coverage to more Americans including those with pre-existing conditions. Other initiatives included improving the health care workforce, public health, Medicare, and access to innovative medical therapies. This act will also benefit oral health prevention education campaigns, as well as create demonstration programs and strength surveillance. Also in March 2010, U.S. Congress passed the Health Care and Education Reconciliation Act, which seeks to improve Medicaid's state funding and Medicare's drug prescription program. Additionally, more funding will go to post-secondary institutions and their students. Support is allocated for general, pediatric, and public health dentistry along with an alternative dental health care provider.

Geographical and Organizational Barriers

GEOGRAPHICAL BARRIERS   Another barrier to access to care is location in terms of geography and organization. A geographic barrier is the distance one is located from providers. This is especially true in rural areas where people may have to travel an hour or more to obtain care. In addition, location is a problem in rural areas because of the lack of a public transportation system, such as bus lines. Some residents of rural areas do not have reliable cars or cannot afford the cost of gasoline. Therefore, an individual must have private means to reach a health care provider. Moreover, the elderly may be incapable of driving a private vehicle or using public transportation and may have to rely on others for transportation.

ORGANIZATIONAL BARRIERS   In addition to geographic barriers, there are also organizational barriers, or lack of available providers. This is especially true in rural areas. The average traveling time in rural districts is estimated to be twice the length of the time in urban districts (Edelman & Menz, 1996). Twenty-five percent of rural residents do not have a dentist available in proximity, and in areas of health care provider shortage, 55% of the population does not have dentists within the same ZIP code area (Knapp & Hardwick, 2000, p. 45).

One study (LeBlanc et al., 1997) reported that in some rural areas, people have to travel as long as three hours to obtain the necessary dental care. This same study reported that 63% of the respondents did not have a dentist in their town, and 45% reported that the nearest dentist was more than twenty miles away. In addition, there was a need to travel in excess of ninety miles to receive care from a dentist who accepted Medicaid. As discussed earlier, there is a problem with dentists accepting Medicaid patients, so there may be providers in a given area that do not accept Medicaid.

Furthermore, some areas have a low ratio of providers to population. An effort has been made by the federal government to provide oral care through the National Health Service Corps (see Box 6-7), through which a health professional may work in an underserved area as part of a

BOX 6-7

Requirements for National Health Service Corps

- Graduate of accredited dental hygiene program at baccalaureate level (4-year)

Or

- Graduate of accredited dental hygiene program at associate level (two-year) and one year of experience

And

- Pass the National Board dental Hygiene Examination

And

- License in state where intending to practice

loan repayment for school. Unfortunately, not many of these positions are available for dental hygienists. And even if a dental hygiene student chooses to work in an underserved area after graduation, this may not be allowed when there is no supervising dentist in that area. An area may not be lacking in dental hygienists but may have no dentists. In that case, the area would not be able to utilize dental hygienists because dentists are needed for the supervision of the majority of dental hygienists.

INCREASING ACCESS   If the supervision laws were to change, dental hygienists would be able to serve more people and increase access to care. This would increase access not only in private-practice settings but also in other areas, such as public health facilities, chronic care facilities, and even schools. For example, access to care for children could be increased if dental hygienists were allowed to perform preventive procedures such as pit and fissure dental sealants without supervision and to bill directly to Medicaid or other insurance plans.

In an effort to help eliminate some of the the disparities and improve access to care, supervision laws have been relaxed (see Chapter 5). Many dental hygienists are making strides to provide preventive oral health care to underserved populations in areas outside traditional private practice and through entrepreneurial opportunities such as school-based, residential care, sealant, homebound, mobile van, Medicaid, and safety net programs (American Dental Hygienists' Association, 2004b; Gutkowski, 2003).

Dental hygienists also participate in clinics and other activities, such as the national Give-Kids-A-Smile Day and the Mission of Mercy events that heighten the awareness of oral health care and provide care on a volunteer basis. Government mandates are being introduced to reduce disparities. For example, some states require elementary schoolchildren to have a dental examination before entrance into schools and at intermediate grade levels (somewhat like the requirement for school physical examinations and vaccinations for school registration and receiving report cards). However, having children's teeth examined does not necessarily mean that the child will receive the needed treatment, and a referral system needs to be in place to make oral health services available and accessible.

At the present time, various levels of oral health care providers are being developed, trained and utilized in the United States. Alaska has sent individuals to New Zealand to be trained as dental therapists, similar to what was developed in Saskatchewan, Canada. Presently, dental health aide therapists are being trained in the state of Washington and will serve the Alaska Native population. Minnesota has passed legislation for both the oral health care practitioner and the advanced dental therapist. The American Dental Hygienists' Association is recommending a master-level dental hygienist, advanced dental hygiene practitioner (ADHP), similar in the hierarchy to the nurse practitioner. More information on these oral health providers can be found in Chapter 9.

Sociological and Cultural Barriers

Even if a person is able to afford care through private or public means and there are providers available, this does not mean that this person will seek the care or have easy access to care. People should not only have the means to obtain dental care but also be motivated to receive care and to recognize the need for such care. Thus, another barrier to access to care is the perceived need for care. Those who do not believe in the importance of oral health and the usefulness of a dental visit would not be willing to access dental care. This is especially true with preventive care. Many individuals do not seek care until they are in pain because they are unaware of the significance of preventive care. However, the availability of a regular provider increases the use of dental services because motivated persons will try to utilize any available services.

DISCRIMINATION   Another sociological barrier to access to care is discrimination. Previous discussion has shown how low-income Medicaid patients are discriminated against by not being accepted by many dentists. Other discriminating factors can be associated with disabilities, and this is against the law. Many practitioners do not feel comfortable or competent with patients who may be mentally or physically disabled; therefore, they may refer them to other providers who have more experience or who are more willing to care for this group of patients. As a result, these disabled individuals may have limited access to care in the vicinity of their homes.

EASING ACCESS   Emphasis on training students to care for disabled patients has been placed in the education curricula of dental and dental hygiene programs in an effort to overcome this disparity and to encourage treatment of disabled individuals in their own vicinity. In addition, oral health care providers are encouraged to treat the disabled, the elderly, the medically compromised, and other special populations in the private-practice setting in order to increase access to care for all individuals. Likewise, some supervision laws for dental hygienists have been relaxed (e.g., from direct supervision to general supervision) so that the elderly or residents in health care facilities can receive preventive dental hygiene care.

LITERACY   The language barrier is another factor that leads to limited access to care. This is especially true with the immigrant population. Newman and Gift (1992) found that ethnic minorities tend to utilize dental care facilities less than those from the ethnic majority. Moreover, immigrants may not know how to seek and obtain the necessary services that will increase their access to care. For example, they may not be aware of public health clinics if the advertisement is geared only to those who speak and read English. The U.S. population is becoming more diverse, and with this comes the need to communicate in a language other than English and to understand and respect cultural differences that relate to health care. Furthermore, even English-speaking citizens may not be able to read educational and instructional materials. Health information should be written at the fifth- or sixth-grade level for the majority of adults and lower levels for those patients at high risk for limited literacy (Weiss, 2003, p. 34). Common terms should be used as opposed to medical and dental terminology and ask the patient to demonstrate or to explain a recommended treatment instead of asking the patient if he or she "understands" a procedure or method of taking medicine.

The population of the United States is shifting. According to the U.S. Census Bureau, it is estimated that the Hispanic population was 15% in 2008, making it the nation's largest ethnic or racial minority, and it will grow to 30% of the population in 2050. There continues to be immigration into the United States, and the Caucasian American will no longer make up the majority of the population. Although non-Hispanic whites make up almost 70% of the population today, they will make up less than 53% in 2050 (U.S. Census Bureau, 2010). People are more likely to seek care from a provider who is of their culture, and providers tend to treat those of their same culture or ethnicity (Geurink, 2005; U.S. Department of Health and Human Services, 2003). One of the reasons for this comfort is that the provider understands and appreciates the culture and respects its beliefs.

In dentistry and dental hygiene, the minority population is not reflective of the number of providers, students, and faculty members. For example, only a small percentage of Hispanics/Latinos, Native Americans/Alaska Natives, and blacks/African Americans were enrolled in dental or allied dental education programs (ADA, 2004) The total enrollment of U.S. dental schools during the 2008–2009 academic year was reported as approximately 60% White, 23% Asian, and 17% other, which includes blacks, Hispanics, American Indians, and unreported (ADA, 2010, p. 26). Over 90 percent (91.5%) of practicing dental hygienists in the United States are non-Hispanic white (ADA, 2009, p. 1). Minority students report a lack of recruitment, retention, and mentoring initiatives to help alleviate this disparity (Lopez, Wadenya, & Berthold, 2003; Veal, Perry, Stavisky, & Herbert, 2004).

CULTURE COMPETENCIES   In addition to increasing the number of minority providers, another way to decrease cultural and ethnic disparities is to raise the awareness of those in practice as well as students. **Culture** is defined as "the inherited ideas, beliefs, values, and knowledge, which constitute the shared bases [basis] of social action" (Hanks, 1986, p. 379). Culture sets the roles and the rules of behavior for a specific group and includes thoughts, beliefs, values, tradition, experiences, customs, rituals, language, practices, courtesies, manners, and relationships (Darby & Walsh, 2010, p. 63; Geurink, 2005, p. 272).

Daniel, Harfst, and Wilder (2008) consider *cultural sensitivity* as an important component of interpersonal communication (p. 69). The importance of *cultural competencies*—understanding and respecting the role of the patient's culture in treatment planning and providing care—is considered in dental hygiene education and practice through accreditation standards, curriculum and competency guidelines, and codes of ethics. Fitch (2004) emphasizes the integration of a patient's culture into dental hygiene care. For example, some ethnic groups are at greater risk for high blood pressure, alcoholism, oral cancer, and diabetes. Other cultures have a high usage of herbal medicine. As discussed in Chapter 3, it is important that the treatment procedures be explained in understandable terms and language; the patient is a partner in dental hygiene care, and autonomy is upheld. One can gain knowledge of another culture, and thus another way to interact with patients and colleagues regarding standards of care and treatment planning, through participation in travel abroad programs where one actually lives and works in an area outside one's own locale (Having & Lautar, 2008) or through Internet-based global classroom activities (Having, Davis, Lautar, & Woodward, 2010).

SERVICE-LEARNING   The education of dental hygiene students mandates working with diverse populations, and opportunities should be available throughout the curriculum. One educational methodology that can improve cultural competence is *service-learning*. Service-learning can be defined as "a structured learning experience that combines community service with preparation and reflection" (Community-Campus Partnership for Health, 2004; Seifer, 1998, p. 273). In order for service-learning to be achieved, the following must be met. First, there must be a need in the community that is met. Second, there must be an increase in academic knowledge or clinical skill that demonstrates a bridge between theory and practice. Finally, there must be a reflective component that fosters critical thinking and good citizenship.

AN EXAMPLE   A school-based sealant program provides needed preventive services to low-income children. In such programs, dental hygiene students place the sealants and thus improve their clinical skill for this procedure and gain experience outside the traditional dental hygiene clinic. They also gain an understanding of those who are "different" from them and learn to reduce barriers that lead to stereotyping, prejudices and disparities. Service-learning can increase cultural competencies by allowing the student to provide services to those in need and not solely to fulfill a clinical requirement. And, depending on how the services are delivered, they may be in a community in which the patient lives, allowing students to experience environments different than their own.

Justice

In Chapter 2, the concept of justice was discussed as an ethical consideration. Justice is a major factor in determining public policy. The allocation of health care resources, including oral health care, is among the prime objectives of public health policies. **Distributive justice** is concerned with how scarce resources are fairly distributed among members of the population. The allocation of resources can be based on the needs of an individual (microallocation) or the public (macroallocation). Distributive justice aims to allocate resources on the basis of equality by rendering treatment facilities open to every citizen equally. It cannot be overemphasized that our society needs and desires to eliminate the obstacles to affordable access to care. Justice should not be overlooked in such a project.

NEED BASED   In addition to the importance of giving equal treatment to every person, treatment should also be based on need. That is, treatment should be given to all people who need it. Factors other than need include contribution and merit. People who are esteemed by society for their distinguished services, efforts, or important contributions may be rewarded with preferential treatment (for a similar discussion, see Darby, 1998, p. 765; Munson, 1996, pp. 38–40). For example, should all individuals be entitled to dental care, and should all dental care be equal? Does everyone have the *right* to the same dental care? Or, is dental care a *need*, and should those most in need have it first?

MERIT BASED   Likewise, is dental care a *commodity*, and should only those who have merit (good qualifications) or the ability to afford the cost have it? The *egalitarian* would believe that equal treatment is a must for everyone. The *utilitarian* would try to allocate resources that would benefit the most while doing the least harm. The *libertarian* may propose that need is not a prime factor in the distribution of resources (Nelson, 2000, p. 580). Others believe that equals should be treated equally and that unequals should be treated unequally. For example, one group of people should have access to costly implants, while other groups can have bridges or partial dentures, each according to its ability to afford the cost.

OTHER CONSIDERATIONS   So the question of which group or individual should get the most expensive and effective alternative raises a problem. Should those who are offered the implants be the ones who have financial resources or higher social position or those who are most valued in society? Should the element of compensation be taken into consideration? For example, should the person who had severe oral injuries as a result of cancer or an accident have a better form of treatment than an individual who lost tooth and bone structures because of periodontal disease due to neglect? A similar question is whether the dental hygienist who has developed carpal tunnel syndrome from dental hygiene practice should be treated for it sooner and at a better level of care than another dental hygienist who developed carpal tunnel syndrome from leisure activities such as playing the piano? Such questions fall in the realm of *compensatory justice,* which is concerned with compensations for wrongs that have been done (Purtilo, 1999, p. 60).

Another form of justice is *procedure justice*, which concerns allocating resources in an orderly and impartial manner. Using the example of carpal tunnel syndrome, if the leisure piano player were first in line for the operation, then the piano player would be operated on before the dental hygienist, who acquired the disease from hard work. There are different views of distributive justice. Although the egalitarian view is the most ethical, it may be the most difficult to apply in practice because of the financial limitations. Yet we should aspire to adopt it as the basis for a better future system of oral health care.

ADVOCACY

Of the five roles of the dental hygienist—clinician, researcher, manager, educator, and advocate—the one role often forgotten is advocacy. At one time there was also the role of change agent, however, that role has been merged with that of consumer advocate. In our dental hygiene education and in our practice settings, emphasis is placed on attaining clinical skills and standards of care, educating our patients, and providing the best treatment available through evidence-based research. For the past few years, pubic health has become the "thread that weaves" these five roles and it provides a great opportunity for dental hygienists to become involved in the advocacy movement for health reform.

Dental hygienists in Canada have divided the competencies for entry-to-practice into two main categories, core abilities and client service abilities. Core abilities are those roles that are shared by other health care providers and include professional, communicator/collaborator, critical thinker, advocate, and manager. Client service abilities are those dental hygiene roles that make dental hygienists specialized and different from other health care providers and include clinical therapist, oral health educator, and health promoter (Sunell, Richardson, Udahl, Jamieson, & Landry, 2008).

ADVOCATING FOR THE PATIENT   Historically, the two professionals that serve as examples of advocates are lawyers and social workers. Lawyers defend and speak on behalf of the accused through the judicial system while social workers facilitate and speak on behalf of the disadvantaged through the social service system. Traditionally, dental hygienists advocate for the profession (Edgington, Pimlott, & Cobban, 2009, p. 270). Usually this was done through dental hygiene associations whose leaders would speak on behalf of dental hygienists in order to move the profession forward with issues such as delegated duties and supervision restrictions. In the clinical settings, dental hygienists have been viewed as advocates of their patients by allowing them to be partners in their care, providing informed consent and education on treatment options and self-care products.

Dental hygienists are becoming more visible as advocates, not only by speaking on behalf of others, but also by doing those actions that will benefit the patient and the general public. Dental hygienists advocate for their patients when facilitating payment from insurance companies and seeking treatment from other oral health specialists. Dental hygienists are increasing their role as advocate through helping the general public have access to oral health that they otherwise would not. For example, dental hygienists are volunteering to provide services such as oral health education and oral cancer screening activities at health fairs, free preventive treatment at annual events targeting the uninsured and underserved populations (i.e., Give-Kids-A-Smile-Day), guidance as to where the disadvantage can seek dental care outside of private dental offices, and speaking at public forums. Dental hygienists are not only seeking employment, but they are creating employment opportunities, that target those populations who otherwise would not have dental hygiene services available to them such as residents in nursing homes, children in schools, and the working poor.

COLLABORATING   Dental hygienists are now being asked to "sit at the table" and become members of coalitions and working groups to improve the health of populations. Partnerships are being developed to change public policy. Thus, dental hygiene is perceived as a stakeholder especially with evidence-based research that links general health with oral health, as well as health becoming a political priority. As a dental hygienist, you may be asked to speak about oral health concerns such as health care reform, fluoridation, access to care, obesity, and other issues where the oral health is a component and your expertise is essential.

Case Study Follow-up #2

In this chapter's case study, who are some individuals or organizations that the dental hygienist can partner with to help meet the oral health needs of children attending this school?

LOBBYING   Being an advocate may involve lobbying, at times referred as social advocacy or political advocacy. Where advocacy is the "act of directly representing or defending others" (Barker, 2003, p. 11), lobbying is influencing a legislator. This can be done by either educating or motivating a political leader, or in some cases, with pay-offs.

Other techniques to inform a legislator about a specific issue include articles or editorials in newspapers, letters, e-mails, phone calls, face-to-face meetings, working on campaigns (simple thing like stuffing envelopes may reap a return favor when you issue comes to vote in legislature), participation in *Lobby* Day, and town meetings.

IMPLEMENTING   One of the best ways to advocate is to speak about an issue either personally to a legislature or at a meeting. A good benchmark to use when talking is to only spend a few minutes about an issue, Knowles and Nocera suggest three minutes (2009, p. 17), while others suggest one minute or so that could be used while waiting in line or riding in the elevator. Encountering a face-to-face meeting, legislators do not have lots of time to spend with you, so give them something to read later about the issue (not long, just quick to read but to the core of the issue) and something to remind them of your visit (i.e., a toothbrush). Remember, you are the expert—speak with credibility and passion, and know your topic and your audience (Jaeks, 2008, pp. 76, 78). Box 6-8 has other ideas on how to advocate.

BOX 6-8

How to Advocate

- Be prepared with facts, not hearsay
- Statistics speak, constituents vote
- One to three-minute statement sets the stage
- Meet face-to-face, do or give something
- Personal stories become community story

Summary

Dental hygiene practice involves social issues that take into account both ethical and legal viewpoints. Three social issues that have legal and ethical ramifications are employment legislation, abuse reporting, and access to care. Patient confidentiality is protected through HIPAA. Dental hygienists are protected in the workplace by legislation; however, the employment laws may not always be applicable to the private dental office, where the majority of dental hygienists work. Dental hygienists need to not only recognize abuse (child, spouse, and elderly) but also help the abused individual through referring and/or reporting to the proper social service or legal authority. Access to care is hindered by financial barriers, location, lack of providers, and sociological factors. Public policy, such as government aid and supervision laws, needs to be changed to increase access to dental hygiene care. Dental hygiene students can increase their awareness of access to care barriers through service-learning activities and development of cultural competencies. Dental hygienists can also participate in advocacy activities for the profession and for the community.

Critical Thinking

1. Divide into groups. Assign each group a different barrier to access to care. Brainstorm ideas that individuals or groups of dental hygienists can do to lessen or eliminate these barriers. Report back to the class.
2. Ask your friends and relatives to state the problems they have encountered in receiving dental or dental hygiene care. What solutions or suggestions are you able to offer to increase their access to dental and dental hygiene care?
3. Write a letter to the editor addressing the barriers to dental and dental hygiene care that you have observed in your community or with the patients you have treated in your program's dental hygiene clinic. Include recommendations.
4. Meet with your legislature to discuss how the dental/dental hygiene practice act needs to be changed to increase access to dental hygiene care for individuals living in your area or for a particular group of individuals who now have limited access to dental hygiene care.
5. Discuss with a partner some of the cultural awareness you have developed through your dental hygiene education through working with other students, patients, or other individuals.
6. Rewrite in simpler language the oral health instructions from a pamphlet usually given to a patient.
7. Write a statement that would take no longer than three minutes to say that would give a legislator some facts and figures about the oral health care of children in a rural area.

CHAPTER 7

Aspects of Practice Management

OBJECTIVES

After reading the material in this chapter, you will be able to

- Discuss the need for practice management in the dental office.
- Identify different *management styles*.
- Differentiate between oral health care and the *business of oral health care*.
- Discuss the *team concept*.
- Identify the benefits of *cross training*.
- Differentiate types of *staff meetings*.
- Differentiate between *employer expectations* and *employee expectations*.
- Identify uses of *public relations* and *image* for the dental/dental hygiene practice.
- Identify *patient needs* as they relate to dental hygiene.
- Discuss how *marketing* relates to the dental/dental hygiene practice.
- Identify advantages and disadvantages of *profit centers*.

KEY TERMS

Accounts payable	Efficacy	Policy manuals
Accounts receivable	Free-rein management	Production
Authoritative management	Huddle	Public relations
Cash flow	Marketing	Team concept
Cross training	Participatory management	

INTRODUCTION

Why is practice management included in the dental hygiene curriculum? The dental practice is also a small business. Understanding how a practice must operate in the business world will assist in that practice's success. Many new graduates are unfamiliar with the everyday operations of the dental practice because they have no experience in a dental office as a dental assistant or staff member. Yet there are numerous tasks to be completed by the office manager, the insurance processor, the dental assistant, and all other staff members employed in a practice.

When employed in multiple practices, the dental hygienist has the opportunity to observe management styles of his or her employer. Many dentists will manage collaboratively with consulting firms, some will hire a full-time office manager, and others may be both the dentist and the manager. However, a team concept is the overall goal for the dental practice because it helps to generate ideas and establish good working relationships with all employees.

Every employee in a practice has a specific job description and role, and many offices will expect employees to help or take over in another area when illness or absence occurs. This chapter is designed to introduce the dental practice as a small business and the many facets to building a team. As a member of the dental team it will be important to understand management styles of employers, the expectations of coworkers, and how the practice sets goals for marketing strategies to increase its success and viability as a business.

Case Study

The practice in which you are currently employed has recently expanded and remodeled with state-of-the-art equipment. This was done partially because of chronic decrease in new patients; annual revenue was not increasing, thus the profitability of the practice was decreasing. Recently, an associate dentist was added who specializes in pedodontics. However, without a steady flow of new patients each month, the dentist will have to let some staff members go. The office has decided to initiate a plan to market the practice, the new associate, and its new environment.

As you read this chapter, consider the following: How would you design a marketing plan that will assist in getting the practice more widely known in the community?

MANAGEMENT CONSULTANTS

Prior to the 1950s, dental students received no practice management information, and today there are still some dental schools that neglect to include it in the curriculum. Dental students are taught theory and technical aspects of saving teeth and restorative dentistry. However, without practice management information, new dentists may be overwhelmed by such tasks as ordering supplies, charging and billing patients, and hiring and firing employees. During the 1970s and 1980s, dental schools began to understand the need to incorporate practice management courses into their curricula. Yet, dental and dental hygiene students are so focused on completing requirements that it is difficult for school curriculum to include enough of this information (Miles, 1999). The assistance of professional management consultants has contributed to an increase in management skills and business knowledge for dental graduates. Dentists and their practices are better prepared to succeed in the business environment.

Consumer-influenced Changes

In the early 1980s, dentistry incorporated more aesthetic and cosmetic procedures as a result of more people keeping their teeth longer and the demand of consumers for "perfect" smiles. This added a new dimension to practice management and how the practice would need to consider marketing strategies. Dentistry is a health care profession, the main goal of which is to provide health care service. However, the dental practice is also a small business that is required to make a profit if it is to survive in the business world. As consumers sought treatment to improve the appearance of their teeth, the practice found that financing was needed along with increased dental insurance processing for preauthorization and billing. Dentists watched **accounts receivable** rise as a result of increasing fees and patients financing their dental work. At the same time, professional management consultants and firms began to capitalize on the need for business skills, knowledge, and operating systems in a dental practice that would increase profitability.

The Focus for Consulting Firms

Many dental practice consultant firms have been around for over 25 years, offering expertise to dentists and their staff and incorporating systems designed to streamline daily tasks while the dental practice realizes a profit. The main objective of consultants is to have all staff members be accountable for their positions. Each member is seen as an important contributor to the team. By training staff to apply business theory, skills, and systems, the overall productiveness of the practice would benefit. Therefore, management consulting firms offered a business approach to operating the dental practice by involving the entire staff and incorporating systems designed to streamline the many tasks that take place on a daily basis.

The use of a professional management consultant or firm may be advantageous to the dental practice and its team members to ensure longevity while providing quality dental care. However, not all management firms or consultants have the "cure-all" solutions to any particular dental or dental hygiene office. When employers make the decision to hire a professional practice management consultant, the consultant requests participation by all staff members. The cost for a professional consultant generally runs high, and the training process may extend over a long period (months to years). The consultant presents ideas and systems that are designed to improve the practice in areas of patient flow, revenue, and overall success. As each practice is trained in these areas, participants can test new ideas in their office and evaluate their success. Employers want to ensure a positive outcome of their investment in the practice. The consultant believes that each staff member has his or her unique responsibilities, resulting in the practice operating more efficiently as each person masters his or her own position. These responsibilities bring accountability to each person for his or her job performance. The consultant introduces specific systems that address different sections or departments of the practice, and the dental team is requested to incorporate them into every operation. The incorporation of computers and software programs have altered many applications performed in the dental office, and it is becoming increasingly necessary for dental professionals to have technical knowledge and skill. These systems are intended to reduce paperwork and establish smooth business operations.

Customized Business Systems

One of the most common drawbacks, as seen by dentists, dental hygienists, and staff members attending management training seminars, is that all the systems designed and promoted by a particular consultant do not fit the organizational or operating structure of the practice. This may be due to the demographic composition of the patients, the numbers of patients seen each day, the specialty of the practice, or other reasons. Sometimes the dentist and the staff decide not to incorporate a particular system because they feel it will not benefit the overall production of the practice. A particular system may complicate a task rather than make it easier and more streamlined. As a result, most dental practices choose to customize their offices by selecting the systems they feel will work more easily and efficiently. A management system customized to the needs of the staff and the practice will more likely be successful and used by all team members. Staff compliance is also likely to be higher. Overall, by selecting systems that best fit the practice, an increase in efficiency and **production** (the amount and cost of services provided to patients per day, week, month, or year) is ensured. When the dental practice operates effectively as a business, patients receive quality care by all those who have participated in making the business successful.

Business and Dental Hygiene

Currently, many states and provinces have begun to allow alternative practice settings, which include rehabilitation facilities, assisted and long-term care facilities, and freestanding dental hygiene practices. Each state or province defines *alternative* or *independent* practice differently, and it is wise to consult with the licensing agency in any specific state or province. The practice of dental hygiene has similar concerns for adding business knowledge as clinicians enter into independent and alternative practice or obtain expanded licensure to include restorative procedures. Billing insurance, collecting fees, managing staff and supplies are among common obstacles that may affect operations and success of the practice. Lack of knowledge in financial management and accounting procedures also hinder success for those who choose this career path.

Although dental schools and dental hygiene programs continue to provide some practice management education for students, the implementation of this knowledge remains a challenge for many practitioners. There are numerous resources available to students and practitioners, such as the American Academy of Dental Practice Administration and specialized publications that focus on practice management issues.

EMPLOYER MANAGEMENT STYLES

As dental hygienists begin a new career, they generally find themselves working in more than one dental office. About 51% of dental hygienists worked part time. Almost all jobs for dental hygienists—about 96%—were in offices of dentists. A very small number worked for employment services, in physicians' offices, or in other industries (Bureau of Labor and Statistics, 2009).

Typically, when dental hygienists choose to work part time, it may be two to three days per week. Consequently, each office will operate differently from the next, and each will expect the dental hygienist to comply with the philosophy of the team and the practice. Leadership in each office may also be unique. Most employees assume that the employer or the dentist is the authority figure and is responsible for making all decisions for the practice and its operations. However, this is not true for all practices. One may find that many employers leave the managing to the receptionist, who may also be the manager. Some practices will have a receptionist and a separate office manager, while others are truly managed by the dentist. Some dental and dental hygiene practices may hire an outside firm to manage all business transactions, such as paying the office bills, billing dental insurance claims, employee payroll, and collecting receivables.

AUTHORITATIVE MANAGEMENT In some dental offices, the dentist makes all the decisions necessary during the daily operations of the practice. This management style is known as **authoritative management**. Auxiliaries carry out the specific requests or orders of the employer. This management style does not allow for staff members to take part in any decisions that may affect them or the duties they must carry out in performing their specific jobs within the practice. Additionally, it does not allow for staff members to feel as though they are part of a team. The dentist in this role may seek to hire employees who are passive in nature so as to avoid any potential conflict in decisions. Authoritative management does not allow for open communication or exchange of ideas that could possibly lead to increased production for the practice and increased patient dental care. Dental hygienists who display confidence and assertiveness may find themselves ill-suited for this type of working environment.

FREE-REIN MANAGEMENT Some dental offices operate as if no one is in a management position. This management style is known as **free-rein management**. Employees may describe the practice as operating in a chaotic environment, as ideas and decisions change on a daily basis. There is no consistency or united direction for the practice. The dentist may appear to have a very relaxed personality and working style, while more than one staff member displays dominant characteristics and leadership. Organization is relatively nonexistent because the dentist and staff have not established short-term or long-term goals for the business. Dental hygienists may find that communication and effectiveness are lacking in this type of environment because of a lack of interest by the dentist and staff to develop specific channels. This system works for them; thus, they see no reason for change. Those who possess high organizational skills may find that they are unable to work effectively in a free-rein environment.

PARTICIPATORY MANAGEMENT The third category of management styles is **participatory management**. As the term implies, all staff members are a part of the decision-making process. This style tends to be advantageous not only for the dentist, dental hygienist, and the staff but also for the patients. Just as management consultants feel that each staff member is valuable in his or her contribution to the practice, so too does participatory management. Each staff member shares responsibility for the decisions and the treatment of patients. Open communication is encouraged, and free-flowing ideas can be exchanged. The employer's objectives are shared by all members in order for the business to be successful. This results in a better working environment for staff, and they are contributing to the longevity of their careers while working toward a common goal.

THE TEAM CONCEPT

Who are members of a dental team? The dentist, dental hygienist, dental assistant, office manager, receptionist, insurance coordinator, and dental laboratory technician are all team members. As previously mentioned, management consultants identify the need to incorporate the entire dental staff to assist in meeting the goals of the dentist and his or her practice. This takes teamwork. Each staff member responsible for accomplishing his or her daily duties also has to be knowledgeable about the duties of all other staff members (see Box 7-1). Thus, the **team concept** was developed.

Team Communication

The office will employ an office manager, a receptionist, an insurance coordinator, and sometimes a dental laboratory technician. Each of these positions will have specific duties designed by the practice. Each office will have personnel for the business, or "front office," whose duties are separate from those of the assistant or dental hygienist working with patients and the dentist in operatories, or the "back office." However, the front office team cannot perform its duties

BOX 7-1

Common Duties of Dental Office Team Members

Team Member Duties

- CPR and continuing education courses
- Collaborating on office policies
- Dentist—licensed professional whose main goal is to improve oral health through
  - Restorative procedures, endodontics, periodontics, orthodontics, oral surgery
- Dental hygienist—licensed professional who performs preventive care and patient education through
  - Nonsurgical instrumentation procedures, patient education, preventive procedures, adjunct therapeutics, and sealants
- Dental assistant—may have a certificate (CDA) or registered (RDA) status and is able to perform expanded functions within the scope of his or her state's dental practice regulations.
- Office staff—may include a receptionist, office manager, insurance manager, or all three who will provide support for the health care providers and patients through managing the everyday operations of the office.

efficiently unless the team working in the back office presents accurate patient information and treatment. Once this information is received, patient billing and insurance claims can be effectively accomplished daily. The same holds true for the dentist, dental assistants, and dental hygienists. The front office team is responsible for scheduling patients and their treatment efficiently to ensure that those in the back office performing treatment procedures can do so without being overworked or running behind schedule. Open communication and understanding by team members of the various aspects of the dental practice will provide for a low-stress, highly productive practice.

DEFINING STAFF ROLES

Each practice that dental hygienists are associated with will likely vary in size and scope of services. For dentists opting to work with a consultant, vision and mission statements are developed to create and provide a common direction for those employed with the practice. If vision and mission statements already exist, rewording may be required to be sure they represent what the practice is really working to accomplish.

MISSION STATEMENT Mission statements are designed to provide philosophical direction to the employees and outline expectations to meet stated goals, and to guarantee quality care to patients. The scope and goals of the practice are often used by the employer to assist in his or her decision for hiring the number of staff members required for the practice to carry out procedures efficiently. Most mission statements are a paragraph in length and use wording that can be applied to the overall practice philosophy for many years.

POLICY MANUALS As mentioned, the goals of the practice often influence the number of office personnel, dental assistants, and dental hygienists to be hired so as to meet those goals outlined by the employer. Most practices will have **policy manuals** that describe the duties of each employee's position (discussed in depth in Chapter 10). It is essential for team members to understand what is expected of them during their association with the practice, as this eliminates confusion about what their job description entails. Each state has specific duties outlined in its dental practice act that describes allowable duties for licensed professionals. All licensed professionals should be aware of the legal duties allowed within their scope of practice. Defining each employee's role will assist in maintaining a smoothly operating practice for the dentist and a better working environment for team members.

CROSS TRAINING

When the employer brings in management consultants, **cross training** is encouraged for all team members. This means that each member in the office will be able to perform the duties of another position in the event of illness or long-term absences, thus eliminating the need to hire a new employee or someone on a temporary basis. Cross training helps maintain the harmony of the office and the efficiency of the business, and patients' treatment can be provided more efficiently as well. The limitation of cross training lies with *licensed* professionals. For example, the certified or registered dental assistant cannot perform the duties of the dental hygienist. However, he or she may be able to assist in procedures that do not require licensed education and training, such as seating and dismissing patients or helping to set up or break down operatories. Furthermore, the dental assistant or dental hygienist may often be asked to perform some front office procedures, such as computer entries, filing, or insurance billing. Dental practices that incorporate such cross-training techniques are able to run more smoothly whenever unforeseen circumstances arise. Do not be surprised when asked to perform such other functions as a part of the team.

STAFF MEETING BENEFITS

Consulting firms and consultants advocate regular staff meetings for dental offices. As a team member, everyone has the responsibility to contribute to improving the daily operations of the business. The frequency and scope of staff meetings will be at the discretion of the employer and his or her team. Many offices find that a monthly meeting is sufficient to exchange information and present new ideas for consideration or implementation. Other offices find they require a weekly meeting. A number of topics may be discussed in staff meetings. Many employers prefer to share the financial portion of the practice so that all employees are aware of what it takes to operate as a business. The staff also has the opportunity to share in the concerns and successes of the business. Open communication plays an important role in the success of not only the business but also those who participate in the team.

Meeting Activities

In general, staff meetings allow all employees to provide valuable information that will benefit each individual and the team collectively. Some topics that may be included for staff meetings are included in Box 7-2.

DAILY MEETINGS Another popular meeting style is the **huddle**. Dental offices that have gone through a professional practice management program have incorporated morning huddles.

BOX 7-2

Common Activities for Team Meetings

- Developing a mission statement for the practice
- Developing office policies with which all members are comfortable
- Understanding the quality and standard of care the practice desires to deliver
- Understanding the business of oral health care delivery
- Setting financial goals for the practice
- Generating and implementing a staff recognition or bonus plan
- Reviewing the daily schedule for changes

During huddles, team members convene for 15 to 30 minutes prior to the onset of each day to discuss pertinent information about scheduled patients and planned procedures. They may also look at scheduling logistics or plan for certain dental assistants to handle certain cases. Huddles also allow the team to prepare possible difficult cases and to set aside time for emergency calls. Additionally, the dentist and the dental hygienist will review the dental hygiene schedule to determine when the dentist is to provide examinations. The morning huddle is beneficial to all team members and sets the stage for a smoothly run, productive day. It also allows for the staff to identify operational strengths and weaknesses on a daily basis.

All of these topics are imperative to the dental practice as a business in order to achieve its goals and realize success. Each team member is essential to the specific duties of the practice and the care provided to patients. When the team incorporates staff meetings and or daily huddles, it provides opportunities to establish and maintain cohesive communications to meet practice goals.

EXPECTATIONS AND PUBLIC RELATIONS

Although the dental hygienist's main task is providing preventive services, the ability to market all services offered to consumers by the practice will be essential in terms of the practice being a small business. As patients become members of a practice, the image represented to them by staff members assists in augmenting the success of the practice.

Employer's Expectations

The dentist must understand the foundation of dental hygiene education and training. Dental hygienists are hired to provide oral health education and dental hygiene procedures. In addition to the foundation of dental hygiene care and treatment there are two key factors in a practice that underlie the clinical aspect: **public relations** and **marketing**. These factors are rarely discussed between employers and employees unless the business has gone through management training and has learned to employ these aspects to enhance its business. The practice is there to serve the public, however, the public may not return if the staff does not represent the dental team in a positive manner. Patients see the dental hygienist and staff as representatives of the practice, both in and out of the office, as does the employer. Appearance, demeanor, and skills are indicative of the overall personality of the business.

IMAGE AND THE CONSUMER   Public relations can involve many aspects of personality, education, and professionalism. As dental hygienists become more comfortable with their new careers, public relation skills will increase to include a broad spectrum of topics. These skills will assist in elevating public opinion of the practice with which the dental hygienist is associated as well as of the dental hygiene profession. Public relations require a variety of programs designed to promote and protect a company's image or its individual products (Kotler, 1997).

Being part of a dental team is being part of a practice. The practice must promote its services to remain a viable business. The dental hygienist's ability to represent himself or herself as a team member and a skilled preventive care specialist is of interest to employers. A confident self-image is how the general public relates to the practice. The role of the dental hygienist becomes important because many patients see hygienists as the experts for preventive oral health care and products designed to improve and maintain oral health.

When beginning to provide oral health care, the dental hygienist is likely to see a patient only once in the first six months of employment. That first impression represents not only the practice but also the employer's ability to select the most compatible person for the business. Thus, public relations and image become an important part of the dental hygiene profession. The astute dental hygienist will use public relations to enhance patient relationships and help improve the understanding of the dental hygiene profession among consumers.

Interpersonal Skills

Some of the skills that will be required to enhance public relations are patience, communication, and empathy. As you gain experience and become more acquainted with patients, you find out some of the concerns they have about dental hygienists. The more common concerns (or complaints) are that dental hygienists are too rough and that they often run behind schedule. Personalities do not always mesh between the dental hygienist and a patient. Interpersonal skills become intertwined with public relations skills. Both are needed to ensure that patients in the practice are comfortable with you as the new professional and that the employer and office management are comfortable that the right decision was made to add you to their team.

PATIENCE   Have patience with your patients. When dental hygienists first begin their career, many may feel as though they should be making gigantic strides toward improved oral health among their patients. This does not always happen, and in fact it could take years before some patients change their habits. Empathy and understanding of each individual will enhance your professional personality and augment your public relations skills. The general public does not always understand how important oral health care is and how it affects total body health or how important dental hygiene education, skills, and career are to the new practitioner. In order to promote the profession and elevate public opinion, dental hygienists find themselves explaining the education and credentials they have for performing the procedures required. It creates ease among the patients treated while increasing their understanding and knowledge of dental hygienists and the dental hygiene profession.

COMMUNICATION   Being able to express ideas and recommendations to patients in a confident, positive manner will enhance their compliance and respect for your professionalism. Negative communication will not be as effective as positive communication skills. Speak to patients as though they were friends or relatives. Efficient home care establishes a positive partnership.

Empathy can be an essential component of effective communication. Empathy means you are able to identify and relate to the patient's feelings, complaints, and concerns. This will be important in gaining patient trust and building rapport on a professional level. Patients must trust their care providers, and your employers need all team members to help build a trusting relationship with the patients, as this gives credibility to the practice as a member in the community.

Communicate Your Education

Few states seek to decrease dental hygiene education, and only Alabama allows what is known as *preceptorship* training (see Box 7-3). It is an advantage for the licensed dental hygienist to also educate patients about the dental hygiene profession. Most dental hygienists hold at least an associate's degree. Many more are going back for a baccalaureate degree, master's degree, or doctoral degree depending on the direction of their career path. Patients do not understand the extent of dental hygiene education and training. You have the opportunity to discuss what is involved in dental hygiene education when employed in private practice and building patient relationships. This also helps to strengthen the image of the practice because patients get a better idea of the dentist's quality staff.

Your Expectations

Just as potential employers have expectations of staff members, so will new graduates when they begin to discuss the duties required in each practice. Dental hygiene students unfamiliar with the operations of a dental practice can benefit by observing a practicing dental hygienist during regular office hours. This may enhance the overall picture of what really goes on in the practice and of a standard schedule for dental hygiene. Another way to gather information on what a practice expects from a dental hygienist is to seek a mentor in the community where you plan to practice after licensure. Determine what you expect from your employer. For example, make your expectation clear:

- Do you expect the employer to purchase new instruments?
- Do you expect the office personnel to schedule your patients?
- Do you expect to have a dental assistant document periodontal probing during your assessment?

BOX 7-3

Dental Hygiene Training through Preceptorship in Alabama

Preceptorship training

Currently, preceptorship training for dental hygiene occurs only in the state of Alabama. Technical training (instrumentation) occurs under the supervision of a dentist in the office versus in a dental hygiene program. Many dental hygienists are active in and supportive of dental hygiene legislation discouraging preceptorship training. For more information, visit the American Dental Hygienists' Association website, key words "preceptorship," and "position papers." (www.adha.org)

By taking the time to list your expectations as an employee, your interview discussion can help set the relationship. Keep in mind that clinical practice is only one aspect of the dental hygiene career. Review the six roles of the dental hygienist in Chapter 8. If you have dental hygiene contacts in other areas, such as in corporate positions, education, or public service, spend some time with those professionals to learn about the numerous options for dental hygiene positions. Spending some time with a seasoned professional in any career setting will allow you to obtain a more comprehensive picture of what occurs when settling into this new career. Depending on what type of employment you seek and obtain, expectations of the employment relationship can be established to insure a collaborative partnership.

Staff Expectations

Staff or team members may perceive the new member as being similar to themselves. They may expect him or her to automatically fall into place and know how the practice operates. Established staff members often forget how disoriented new employees are when it comes to finding supplies and equipment. The office manager and front office staff may have expectations similar to the employers'. They may expect that the dental hygienist will be open to making phone calls and confirming appointments or filing patient charts if there is downtime. The office may be under the assumption that the dental hygienist is willing to assist in ordering supplies and putting them away as they are received. As a team member, it is important to remember that everyone in the practice has the same goal: to work together productively to provide quality dental care. This also may mean that everyone is open to helping out in other departments in order to maintain scheduling demands.

These are examples of why you want prepare questions regarding the job description for each interview you choose to pursue. It is important to understand the daily operations of the office and what has been the general operation in the past with former employees and dental hygienists. Decreasing the possibility of first-day jitters or mistakes is essential to making a good first impression with new coworkers and the patients seen that first day.

Patient Expectations

Being the new person is one part of employment that many can relate to. Patients of an established practice are savvy to new faces, high staff turnover, and negative atmospheres in the office. Patients expect that the dental staff, whether new or not, are experienced in all aspects of treatment procedures, materials, equipment, and operations.

There is a period of adjustment in every new position. The dental hygienist must learn the location of materials, equipment, and supplies while learning the equipment. He or she must also learn charting systems, computer systems, and appointment policies, and may also need to become familiar with how services are charged and billed to insurance companies. Practitioners who are replacing someone who just retired from the practice will want to orient patients to themselves and their dental hygiene philosophy. For some patients, change may not be easy, and their comfort becomes important.

This is essential in initiating a new professional relationship. Most often, the new dental hygienist will inform patients that he or she is new to the office and still learning the location and operations of the practice. This information helps the patient understand if the practitioner takes more time than usual to complete a procedure or if he or she must stop treatment to ask coworkers for assistance. The more information given to the patient, the more at ease both parties will be during this important first impression. Coworkers and patients are there to assist in the orientation to a new environment; however, be open to learning how the practice operates.

As mentioned, public relations deal with image. How the public, the dental community, and the patients view the practice, the staff, and the practitioners is important to maintaining the longevity and reputation of the practice. Building skills for public relations such as interpersonal skills will contribute greatly toward the image of the dental hygienist and the practice.

Case Study Follow-up #1

Determine some public relations or image ideas that may benefit in building patient relationships.

MARKETING AND THE DENTAL PRACTICE

Dental practices find that marketing will assist in growing their business from several aspects. Many times a marketing campaign will focus on the dentists' specialty such as dental implants, orthodontics, and cosmetic dentistry. Through successful advertising strategies, the marketing campaign will bring new patients to the practice. Other types of marketing might include targeting the elderly population using prosthetic dentistry or non-orthodontic procedures using products like Invisalign appliances. Whether a practice is new or well established, the dentist may have the need to market in order to enhance and maintain growth.

Marketing is also defined as a social and managerial process by which individuals and groups obtain what they need and want through creating, offering, and exchanging products of value with others (Kotler, 1997). Those who seek care in a dental office are fulfilling a need: dental care. Marketing also targets human wants and demands. Wants are desires for specific items that will satisfy the need. Demands are wants for specific products. This means the practice must use marketing techniques to offer its product and services. Marketing is one of the keys to maintaining a successful practice and includes planning and management.

Often, in larger practices a marketing and business manager may be employed to coordinate many factors of a marketing plan chosen by the employer. For example, it could be the most advanced materials used for restorative procedures or the latest technology for diagnostic and assessment procedures, such as intraoral cameras and digital radiology. Thus, there is an exchange of goods or products to meet the needs of both the practice and the patient; consumers exchange money for services and procedures performed by the dentist, dental hygienist, and staff. So how does marketing relate to the dental hygienist?

Using Expertise to Market the Practice

Recall the dental materials course during dental hygiene education. During that education, students learned properties of materials and techniques for restorative procedures. Patients who frequent the practice and have regular dental hygiene visits are apt to question the dental hygienist on the latest technology or seek advice on the best and latest dental care products. Addressing these questions for the consumer is how the practice markets its services. All staff should be knowledgeable about their specific areas of expertise and should know who in the practice can provide answers to questions they are unsure of. The dentist is likely to contribute to continuing education for licensed employees by including them in courses that promote the latest materials or technology. For licensed professionals, there may be requirements by your state to accumulate

BOX 7-4

The Value of Marketing a Practice

1. The market is constantly changing.
2. People forget.
3. Marketing strengthens identity.
4. Marketing helps to retain long-term patients.
5. Marketing gives patients and staff motivation.

Source: "The Vital Role of Practice Marketing," Connie Hazel (1998).

a certain number of continuing education units per year or license cycle. Dentistry is a science, and science continues to find improvements for numerous human needs. The more information and education the staff members have on materials, procedures, and techniques, the greater the opportunity to expose patients to procedures that may be of interest to them.

Successful Marketing

When patients are satisfied with the service and with the result of their treatment, the practice sees increased production and revenue (see Box 7-4). Satisfied consumers tend to refer family and friends who may seek the latest techniques and materials for restorative services. Marketing skills of the staff become an essential portion of the practice and another area of practice management that underlies the delivery of quality dental care.

Changes in market occur when patients move away as well as when new families move into an area. Marketing will ensure that both longtime residents and newcomers are aware of the dental practice. Insurance companies also cause market change as they become more restrictive, limiting dental care options for some patients. If the practice stops promoting itself and its services—accommodating, where possible, changes in insurance programs—it may see a decrease in patient flow and referrals.

Using Advertising

Advertising assaults us on a daily basis and in a tremendous way. Radio, television, print advertising, and social networking websites are the primary means by which companies get their messages to us, and they send their messages over and over again—because people forget. Businesses must maintain a public presence, usually through advertising, in order to retain clientele. Many dental offices rely on word of mouth to increase their patient base. While word of mouth is effective, it is limited in its market reach. Through advertising, a practice can reach thousands of existing and potential patients, strengthening its identity and assuring consumers that it is here to stay. Retaining long-term patients is as important as attracting new patients to a practice. Patients generally frequent a practice because of the service they receive and the professionalism of the staff. A practice must also remain progressive, keeping up with the latest procedures and technologies, so that patients are assured that they will continue to receive the most modern care available. A practice should promote its advanced services in its marketing strategies. Both patients and staff can be motivated by effective marketing. Working in an office that is well known in a community elevates the staff morale, and patients are reassured in their choice of a quality practice for their dental care.

Marketing the Patient's Health Care

Patients seek dental care because of a need. That need comes in different forms. Michele Darby and Margaret Walsh (2003) have identified 11 human needs (see Box 7-5) as they relate to dental hygiene care. These will be important for you as a preventive care specialist, as will an understanding of the exchange of goods (money) and services (treatment):

When patients seek dental care, they are attempting to fulfill one need or a combination of needs. A marketing strategy is able to target specific services that fulfill these needs for consumers. All staff members are expected to be knowledgeable in the materials and techniques that are on the cutting edge of dental care, as this area is also of interest to many patients. These are only a few reasons for maintaining licensure with continuing education courses. For the dental hygienist, patient needs assist in designing treatment and home care programs for maintaining quality dental hygiene care. Patients want integrity and compassion from their caregiver. Patients want to be assured that they are receiving the best their dollar can buy. Possessing competent marketing skills will help in that assurance.

Marketing the Practice

Dentistry and dental hygiene care have changed dramatically over the past 25 years. There was a time when patient treatment focused on "fixing" whatever ailment the patient complained of. Prevention was not the basis of oral care. Since then, patient care has changed, and the delivery aspect of that care has seen a dramatic transformation. Dental practices need a positive patient

BOX 7-5

Basic Human Needs

- Safety—freedom from harm or danger
- Freedom from pain/stress—exemption from physical and emotional discomforts
- Wholesome body image—positive mental representation of one's own body
- Skin and mucous membrane integrity of the head and neck
- Nutrition—the need for a balanced diet
- A biologically sound dentition—need for intact teeth and restorations that provide function
- Conceptualization and problem solving—to grasp ideas and make sound judgments
- Appreciation and respect—need for acknowledgment and achievements
- Self-determination and responsibility—need to exercise firmness of purpose about one's self and behavior
- Territoriality—to possess a prescribed area of space or knowledge
- Value system—freedom to develop one's own sense of importance

Source: Darby & Walsh, 2003.

base and **cash flow** to maintain existence in the business world. The practice may focus on creating a niche or may target a particular market that helps it stand out as a leader in dental services within the community. The business may opt to convert its delivery systems to include those of the latest technology. Technology may include modern equipment, computer programs, digital radiology, lasers, and caries detection. These things can result in higher patient volume and perhaps increased patient referral.

The practice must analyze what it currently offers in the way of programs that could draw more consumers. After identifying their strengths and weaknesses, the practice can then rely on staff members to market the best programs directly to the patients. Offering them the service that will fulfill their need—the reason they sought service in the first place—is the first and easiest step when patients are physically in the office. Marketing the practice takes a lot of energy and planning. Many employers will seek professional consultants to focus on the direction the practice or staff may want to pursue. For example, many offices have opted to focus on cosmetic dentistry. Others find they do better at providing family, implant, or other specialty services. Finding a specific niche in the oral health care field means the practice must target its own talents.

Marketing dental hygiene means the practice and the dental hygienist must target patient education on the profession and the professional and its important role in total systemic health. Marketing aids the employer, the staff, and the practice in focusing on specific programs that have been chosen to provide to its patients. The overall outcome will result in a profitable business.

Marketing Yourself

Along with public relations and the image the dental hygienist presents to the employer, staff, and patients, new practitioners will also become adept in marketing the practice, techniques, materials, and services. Dental hygienists have to market themselves every day. Patients need to know that the dental hygienist is a professional oral care specialist. Many patients see their dental prophylaxis as just a cleaning. Most often, dental hygienists encounter patients who are unaware of what a prophylaxis involves, as well as procedures like root planing. Additionally, patients are unaware that it may take four years to get through a dental hygiene education. Even 2-year dental hygiene programs require a number of years of prerequisite education. Consumers are unaware of the spectrum of dental hygiene knowledge. They are unaware of what it takes to maintain a license through continuing education. These are reasons why marketing becomes an important aspect of dental hygiene. Patients need to understand that the person providing these services is in tune with the latest techniques and materials. Because of continuing education, the dental hygienist will have the ability to provide information patients are seeking. Ultimately, dental hygienists are marketing themselves and all the knowledge acquired over many years. Everything learned is applied to everyday working environments. Patient questions often require marketing skills that allow the dental hygienist to be the professional consumers want as a care provider.

Marketing Strategies

Other strategies that may be advantageous to the practice and the dental hygienist as a professional will include programs and activities that can bring attention to the practice and help shape it as a leader in the community. Some examples that can be used to increase public exposure for the office:

- Become sponsors for local events or organizations, such as children's sports teams, soccer, baseball, and swimming teams. It might also include sponsoring local health fairs and school events.

- Contribute oral health articles to the local newspaper.
- Appear on the local television or radio stations to promote National Dental Hygiene Month (October) or other nationally and locally recognized days.
- Participate in presenting continuing education courses designed for colleagues as well as other health care providers (e.g., nurses' aides, nurses, home health aides).
- Offer free oral cancer screenings in the month of October.
- Organize a Dental Health Day when all services to children are free.
- Volunteer, as an office, for a community service project.

As a member of one's own professional organization, volunteering becomes second nature in promoting oral health.

Marketing and Profit Centers

Profit centers are another way for the practice to increase its productivity. Profit centers consist of specific products that are offered to patients from within the office. In today's modern dental practice, it can be easy to implement a profit center that not only results in revenue over and above standard dental procedures but also allows for increased compliance among the patients and may set the practice apart from others in the community. There are advantages and disadvantages of profit centers and possible ethical and legal aspects that may need to be addressed by the practice's business manager and accountant.

Profit Centers and Patient Compliance

As the dental hygienist, your interest lies in getting patients to comply with the recommendations you have prescribed for them so that they maintain better oral health. Most profit centers focus on patient needs and compliance. The most popular patient need (or, rather, demand) is teeth whitening or bleaching. This is an easy avenue for the practice to offer a procedure that falls in the latest technology category, fulfills the need (or desire) of the patient, and results in additional income for the practice. Therefore, the practice can set up displays that promote teeth whitening. For example, it may use before-and-after photos of its patients. Additionally, the practice may have its entire staff whiten their teeth. Now the staff is able to describe the procedure to the interested patient from firsthand experience.

For patient compliance, the practice typically finds that it can easily focus on products that are recommended by the dental hygienist. These products may be oral irrigation devices, electric toothbrushes, or therapeutic dentifrices. These products are easily acquired by the office from the manufacturer and offered to the patient for purchase. Many times, the key marketing tool is convenience. Dental hygienists often recommend certain products because of their **efficacy** or patient acceptance. Patients are apt to purchase the recommended product because it is conveniently located in the office. This too creates additional income for the practice.

Profit Center Options

Other profit centers include halitosis clinics and products and soft-tissue management programs. Halitosis clinics address patients with chronic bad breath. During oral hygiene education courses, students learn that bad breath usually results from bacteria and periodontal disease. However, there are many other reasons, some of which include medications, systemic diseases, and reasons that dentists and professionals cannot diagnose. As a result of this increasing patient need, halitosis clinics have opened throughout the country. The office can purchase specialized equipment and products known as volatile sulfur compounds specifically developed for causes of halitosis. Once the diagnosis is made, patient compliance will be higher when the product can be purchased in the office. Here again is an example of addressing a patient need while marketing a unique service that makes the office stand out from other practices. Soft-tissue management programs are another specialized area for profit centers. These programs are based on the patient's need to improve oral health due to periodontal diseases and pocket depth. Weekly visits are required for dental hygiene treatment as well as patient education and modification. Patient education includes miniclasses. For example, the dental hygienist educates the patient on how to manage oral health using an electric toothbrush and other products combined with frequent professional treatments. Many practices today have soft-tissue management protocol and laser procedures to offer patients. As the dental hygienist, you may be expected to participate in or design such a program.

Other Practice Considerations

Disadvantages for profit centers may include ethical and moral issues, not to mention legal issues. Ethically, is the practice allowing autonomy? By making certain products available to patients, is the business allowing them to make the choice that is best for them? The practice cannot afford to bring in every type of product on the market. Therefore, the dentist and the dental hygienist can select products with long-term proven success to overall improved consumer oral health. Does this limit the consumer's decision? Should the consumer be allowed to see all products before purchasing a specific model or item? The moral aspect is twofold. The practice believes it is providing a convenience to its patients, yet it is making a profit based on sales. What is the true motivation for including a profit center?

As professionals, most dental hygienists prefer not to "sell" dentistry or dental hygiene. The questions are not easily answered, and the dental hygienist will want to feel comfortable and confident that the reasons for a particular profit center fall in line with his or her professional philosophy. Legally, the practice needs to be sure that revenues from sales items are taxed appropriately, if required by state or federal regulations, for retail sales. This will require consultation with a tax consultant.

Profit centers are increasing in today's dental office, and it is one way to keep the patient healthy while making the practice unique. The dental hygienist can be an integral part in creating profit centers that address patient needs. Both public relations and marketing play a role in making the practice you work in profitable and successful in the eyes of the consumer. Being a part of the dental hygiene profession will bring a variety of aspects to your new career, increasing the spectrum of knowledge you bring to your patients every day.

Case Study Follow-up #2

Using the information from marketing strategies and how a practice can focus on growing the business, discuss some strategies that are more commonly used for a general dentistry practice.

Summary

Although the dental practice provides dental care, it is also a small business and must realize a profit to remain a viable source of income for all those who are employed by the practice. The 1980s saw a surge of consultants and consulting firms targeting the dental practice. Many consultants have succeeded in incorporating systems that streamline the daily tasks performed in the dental office. However, not all systems fit easily into every dental practice. Usually, the dentist and his or her team customize the systems to be incorporated. Dental hygienists are typically employed in more than one dental office. Management styles will vary in each practice setting. Authoritative management indicates that the dentist is the decision maker. This does not allow for other staff members to present ideas that may benefit the practice and their working environment. Free-rein management may mean the office operates in a chaotic state, as the authority figure or decision maker cannot be identified. Communication channels have not been identified, as the staff has not seen the need to design such channels. Participatory management implies participation from every staff or team member in the office. Each individual takes an important role in the development of the working environment and the success of the practice. Communication lines remain open and encourage the exchange of ideas. Defining staff roles decreases potential confusion as to who is responsible for certain tasks in the office. Most practices have developed policy manuals to achieve complete understanding of each staff member's roles. Management consultants advocate cross training, as this will maintain smooth operations during staff illnesses or long-term absences. After the dental practice undergoes management training with a professional consulting firm, staff meetings or huddles may be incorporated at intervals determined by the dentist and his or her team members. Implementing regular meetings encourages the team members to plan their day so that it runs smoothly. In addition to daily planning, exchanging ideas for practice development may enhance the overall goals and objectives for the business. Public relations and marketing are two aspects of the dental practice that underlie meeting the needs and demands of the general public. Public relations deal with the image of the practice, the dentist, and its staff members. Employers rely on staff members to represent and promote the practice to patients as they are treated in the office. This promotes the word-of-mouth advertising needed to remain a viable community business. Staff members market technology, procedures, and materials to patients. Those who frequent the practice are seeking to fulfill a need or demand. Marketing deals with the exchange of products to fulfill a need. Marketing the ability of the practice to meet those needs is what the employer expects. Continuing education helps keep the staff members current on the latest trends in dentistry and dental hygiene procedures. Marketing targets specific human needs. Human needs have been identified as they relate to dental hygiene. Other reasons for marketing are that people move, people forget, and marketing can help to retain long-term patients. Profit centers are a way to increase practice revenue while increasing patient compliance. The dental hygienist can be instrumental in creating a profit center, using products and home care appliances recommended to patients. Profit centers targeting tooth whitening, halitosis, and home care products are more popular and widely accepted by patients.

Critical Thinking

1. Identify the management style in a practice in which you would like to practice. Explain why you chose this particular style? How does it fit with your personal philosophy?

2. Briefly explain why not all systems recommended by a management consultant may work in every practice.
3. Explain the purpose of the team concept and why this is essential in practice.
4. List some topics that may be included during staff meetings or morning huddles. How does this influence the interaction between team members?
5. Identify some of the expectations that were discussed in a past interview and some of the expectations that were not discussed yet were realized after beginning the job.

6. Using a local telephone book, look at some of the advertisements for dental offices in your area. Identify terms used in the advertisement that promote the image of the practice.
7. If you were asked to set up a profit center, what type would you select, why, and how would you set it up? Be as detailed as possible.
8. Identify marketing techniques used by local dental offices in your community.

CHAPTER 8

The Business of Dental Hygiene

OBJECTIVES

After reading the material in this chapter, you will be able to

- Describe the scope of the *dental hygiene diagnosis* as it relates to building a practice.
- Discuss *business* aspects for dental hygiene.
- Discuss *time management* issues and plan a treatment hour.
- Identify *leadership* traits.

KEY TERMS

Advanced appointment
    system
Capitation
Dental health maintenance
    organization
Dental hygiene assessment

Dental hygiene diagnosis
Health maintenance
    organization
Mail system
Overhead
Preauthorization

Preferred provider
    organization
State assistance
Usual, customary, and
    reasonable

INTRODUCTION

Dental hygienists have a primary duty to assess the oral health of their patients. Recall the core values of beneficence and nonmaleficence discussed in Chapter 2. Both terms relate to benefiting the patient. Thorough assessment and treatment planning is not only essential to the benefiting the patient, it also essential in working collaboratively within the dental practice. The dental hygiene assessment or diagnosis may be required for submitting documentation to an insurance company. Preauthorization may be required prior to beginning treatment. Determining the length and interval of appointments helps establish a varied daily schedule, which contributes to the overall production goals for the practice. This chapter discusses how the dental practice must operate in order to maintain viability and success, balance treatment procedures, dental insurance procedure codes, practice goals, and daily scheduling.

As an employee in the practice, the dental hygienist will learn how to manage time wisely and work with other practitioners. Many dental hygienists are responsible for scheduling their own patients; thus, having a good understanding of production goals and varying procedures aids in maintaining a daily schedule that is manageable. Additionally, as graduates are likely to begin careers in private practice, there are opportunities to begin thinking about alternative career paths as a dental hygienist, this chapter briefly introduces other roles for consideration and career longevity.

Update: As of January 2009, the American Dental Associations' Commission on Dental Accreditation modified dental hygiene education standards and the phrase "**dental hygiene diagnosis**" and replaced the term and intent with "assessment." During formal education, students engage in patient assessment, which leads to the etiology of current oral conditions and designing and implementing a treatment plan. Although the term has been replaced, dental hygiene programs have not changed the way students are taught to assess the etiology of gingival and periodontal disease and treatment plan for optimal patient care.

In March 2010, the American Dental Educators Association approved a resolution in support of a dental hygiene diagnosis definition as included in the competencies developed for dental assisting, dental hygiene, and dental laboratory technicians: The dental hygiene diagnosis is an overall component of the dental diagnosis. It is the identification of an existing or potential oral health problem that a dental hygienist is educationally qualified and licensed to treat. The dental hygiene diagnosis utilizes critical decision-making skills to reach conclusions about the patient's dental hygiene needs based on all available assessment data.

Case Study

You have been working in private practice for 15 years. Recently, there has been an influx of corporate-owned dental clinics that accept Medicaid and preferred provider organization (PPO) insurance plans. One of these offices is seeking a dental hygienist with experience in how a practice operates because the owners are businessmen, not dentists. They will also be hiring dentists. You have applied for the position and have an appointment for an interview. Identify leadership traits in yourself and what you can bring to this position. How will you lead staff and dental professionals?

As you read this chapter, consider the following: Leadership qualities are beneficial to healthcare providers. What qualities do you feel you already have that can help get those you may supervise on board with the vision you have for this practice as it services families who are economically challenged?

DENTAL HYGIENE ASSESSMENT

Dentists diagnose dental disease in general, such as carious lesions and their extent, in order to determine causes and recommend treatment that will remedy the condition. The main concerns for dentists are treating the symptoms, preventing new and recurrent caries, and reconstructing lost dentition. As you learned during your dental hygiene education and applied in your clinical training, the **dental hygiene assessment**, or "process of care," serves a completely different purpose than the dental diagnosis. It focuses on problems or potential problems related to oral health and disease versus dental disease (Darby & Walsh, 2003).

Thorough Patient Assessment

Licensed dental hygienists are responsible for identifying the deficient human need as related to dental hygiene. Identifying a possible etiology and designing and planning treatment in order to remedy the patient's condition is the goal of each practitioner. As a professional, you will also have to deal with patients' perceptions, beliefs, and attitudes, and this requires interpersonal skills and obtaining factual information. Other factors must also be considered if professional services are to be successful. These factors may include the following:

- Recognizing the causes (etiology) that resulted in poor oral health
- Identifying the human need the patient is seeking to fulfill
- Assessing patients' records, such as medical and dental histories
- Recognizing abilities or inabilities of the patient to comply with your recommendations
- Prioritizing dental hygiene treatment, recare, and maintenance

Assessment, dental diagnosis, evaluation, implementation, and interpretation are intertwined when it comes to helping patients fulfill a need. Ethically, licensed practitioners are required to use these skills to determine oral health deficits and provide the best treatment. For example, patients are typically eager and expect the dental hygienist to provide them with interpretive results of radiographs. Yet legally, the dental hygienist cannot diagnose dental disease. However, recall the human needs as related to dental hygiene identified by Darby and Walsh. Using that information, the clinician is now able to identify the human deficit as it relates to the patient's oral hygiene, which is the need for sound dentition. Therefore, after evaluating new radiographs and observing a carious lesion, the dentist can be informed prior to his or her oral examination. Why? Because the patient's need for sound dentition has been identified as the deficit. Generally and legally, a final dental diagnosis is always determined by the dentist.

The process for the dental hygiene assessment includes other factors worthy of discussion. As defined, examination of symptoms and analysis of facts are required before finalizing results. The astute dental hygienist will gather the appropriate data using the medical and dental history along with current information provided by the patient. Using this information, clinicians are able to look for patterns or a series of patterns that assist in developing possible etiologies for the patient's current oral health. Assessment takes quality evaluative skills and application of the knowledge gained in dental hygiene school as well as information from continuing education courses.

Building and Perfecting Skills

Licensed practitioners will want to continuously build and perfect assessment skills as they gain experience in the clinical setting. In doing so, the chance of misevaluation will decrease, and patients will benefit from the clinician's expertise. Another immediate resource of expertise is the employer. The dentist is available for consultation about patients each day. Working as a team, the staff can ensure that patients in the practice receive quality dental health care.

In dental hygiene education, students may have learned to use terminology that does not specifically lead to diagnosing dental disease, such as *suspicious, signs of,* or *area of concern.* These terms and phrases do not designate dental diagnosis or dental hygiene diagnosis; they simply assist the professional in informing the patient of his or her present condition.

Another example of dental hygiene assessment is the clinical evaluation of existing restorations. On evaluation of restorations, a margin that is faulty and possibly causing recurrent decay may be identified. This would meet the criteria for needing sound dentition and restorations that function. So what is the dental hygienist's responsibility? Using the process for the dental hygiene assessment, the practitioner can determine that restorations will need to be replaced. The dentist and the patient will discuss the best dental treatment option; however, as the dental hygienist, you can inform your patient that a defect in the existing restoration is present and that treatment may be required.

Preventative and Home Care

Using practiced assessment skills, dental hygienists focus on problem areas. The basis of preventive treatment is being able to determine the etiology behind current oral hygiene conditions so that modifications are implemented. Patient compliance is an area the clinician targets when evaluating for the most effective home care recommendations. Patients often complain that their dental hygienist reprimands them every time they have a dental prophylaxis. Can you imagine what it might be like if the patient sees a new dental hygienist who is unfamiliar with his or her oral health history? During dental hygiene education, make an effort to look for the positive aspects in patients and the successes they have achieved. Look for strengths in patients and take advantage of them when discussing home care. Everyone wants to be praised for his or her accomplishments. Otherwise, no one would attempt to make improvements. Patients want to be treated by someone who sees their strengths, not their weaknesses. Interpersonal skills become imperative when discussing these aspects of oral health.

Examples such as these display what is involved in the diagnosis process. Ethically, the clinician must determine the oral health deficit and inform patients. The dental hygiene assessment assists the preventive care specialist to present accurate information to the patient so that the patient has the opportunity to participate in his or her oral health care. It is a valuable tool for the dental hygienist. Use it for processing patient information prior to designing a treatment plan, recare, and maintenance. Each patient is an individual, and each dental hygiene diagnosis and treatment plan is customized to that individual's needs. The dental hygiene profession is unique and rewarding for many who choose this career. Each patient, each case, and each dental hygienist is unique and should be viewed and treated with that uniqueness in mind.

MAXIMIZING SKILLS

In Chapter 7 you identified and defined public relations and marketing skills. The dental hygienist must be able to recognize his or her own limits in their assessment and instrumentation skills. New graduates may be hesitant to realize at the start of their new career that they are challenged to perform the required procedures on cases they have just treatment planned. Instrumentation skills are still relatively new, and new hygienists are used to having instructors at their side. Be careful about marketing skills that have yet to be fully developed. Those with experience realize their limits and skills and know that a specialist will better serve his or her patients. As a team member, a hygienist has professional resources available: the employer and the professional community he or she has developed while providing patient services. Dental hygienists will have many of these resources at their disposal. At the beginning of a new career, review strengths and weaknesses in clinical abilities and knowledge:

- Be honest about how much time is needed for appointments while gaining speed and familiarity with the new position.
- Understand how the practice handles complex cases. Consult with the dentist and other dental hygienists in the practice about when patients are referred to the specialist.
- Discuss which type of treatment cases will be scheduled with the experienced dental hygienist and which will be scheduled for you.
- As you gain experience with the practice, meet with employer to discuss progress and added responsibilities.

Numerous aspects become incorporated into the development of a dental hygiene professional. For example, most dental hygienists obtained at least 4 years of formal education. Many have been exposed to the scientific background of dental hygiene theory, practice, dental materials, and technology. Some have gained knowledge about public relations, marketing, and interpersonal communication. And each will be continuously exposed to educational courses that are applicable to his or her licensure and interests. How does this apply to each dental hygienist and his or her patients?

By using expert resources and specialists, preventive care specialists are better serving the overall health of patients. This expansion of expertise allows each to exercise critical thinking and evaluative skills. Recall the meaning of beneficence: doing what will benefit or help a person or patient. Maximizing your clinical and intellectual skills will insure doing the best you can for patients.

Case Study Follow-up #1

Can you identify strengths and weaknesses in your clinical skills as you prepare for licensure? How might you approach your weaknesses in a new position?

Keep in mind some of the ideas on how to build and maximize clinical and critical thinking skills as you read on to the leadership section.

DEVELOPING LEADERSHIP QUALITIES

Oftentimes the dental hygienist is asked to take a leadership or management role by overseeing dental hygiene production, supplies, appointments, and perhaps personnel. Since the dental office operates as a business, a good leader will contribute to the sustainability of a successful bottom line. Not everyone is cut out to be a leader or manager. This, too, is important to identify. It can assist in determining who the real leader might be among those in the practice. When employed in more than one dental practice, the dental hygienist has the opportunity to observe leadership or management styles in their employers, as described in Chapter 7. Recognizing leadership traits within yourself is important for success as a dental hygienist and can enhance relationships with employers and coworkers. There are many definitions and descriptions of "leadership," so for the purpose of this text we will use the following definition, which focuses on the key qualities most commonly used to describe leadership:

Leadership is a process whereby an individual influences a group of individuals to achieve a common goal (Northouse, 2007, p. 3). Managers are not the same as leaders, yet these terms are often used interchangeably. Understanding their differences can help you succeed in either role.

MANAGERS Managers have an authoritative role over others, yet the ultimate goal of the manager is to make sure everyone has done his or her job in order to obtain specific results. Managers may oversee one or more subordinates and are accountable to a supervisor. Managers may or may not be held responsible for the work done by their subordinates; therefore, many times the quality of work can be adversely affected as personal investment may be lacking. Managers may develop leadership skills over time based on the many situations that occur while in the role.

LEADERSHIP On the other hand, leadership may be described best as an influential relationship with subordinates or coworkers where the outcome of a project resulted in significant change. Leadership is noncoercive and based on relationships where there is a mutual purpose or goal (Rost, 1993, p. 103). Table 8-1 is a small example of the different traits in how a leader and manager will interact with subordinates or followers based on the subject or situation.

It takes patience and diligence to become an effective leader: promote strengths and work on improving weaknesses. The team leader is also a team member. When the dental hygienist is asked to take more responsibility in the practice, becoming a good leader can enhance the many roles available in the profession. Take a leading role by first identifying leadership traits you already hold and expanding on those that will benefit your leadership style.

TABLE 8-1 Traits in Leadership versus Manager

Situation	*Leadership Traits*	*Manager Traits*
Focus of the One in Charge	**Leading People**	**Managing Work Done**
Decisions	Facilitates a collective decision	Makes the decision
Power	Personal charisma is viewed as confident	Formal authority is followed from the top
Style	Transformational: changes and transforms others	Transactional: exchanges things of value to advance agendas
Wants	Achievement of others	Results produced by others
Risk	Takes them to achieve the goal	Minimizes them and follows the rules
Rules	Breaks them to induce ideas	Makes them to avoid consequences
Conflict	Uses conflict to improve relationships	Avoids conflict to keep workers focused on their job
Concern	What is right for all those involved	Being right is important for managing others
Credit	Gives credit to the entire team	Takes credit for the work done by the team
Blame	Takes blame when things go wrong	Blames others when things go wrong

Adapted from: Leadership vs. Management http://changingminds.org (2002–2009).

Case Study Follow-up #2

After reading about leadership qualities, which do you identify in yourself? How can these qualities better assist you in your practice or your career?

THE BUSINESS OF DENTAL HYGIENE

Profitability in the dental hygiene department is one important factor many employers frequently review. There are those employers who believe that dental hygiene loses revenue, while many others believe that dental hygiene is the pulse of the practice. However, employers may not realize the revenue referred back to them by their dental hygienists when faulty restorations or new carious lesions have been identified during patients' semiannual prophylaxis, not to mention the numerous patients who are seeking cosmetic improvements with their dentition and smile. Instead, they may see only the outgoing salary and possible benefits the dental hygienist "costs" the practice.

Overhead Costs

Dental practices may view their hygiene department as just that: a department. This means that **overhead** costs need to be considered and monitored, as does the amount of production the dental hygienist can produce given daily, weekly, and monthly scheduled procedures. What can a dental hygienist produce? Recall the meaning of production: the total cost of procedures performed over a given period. Table 8-2 gives an example of what a typical day might entail based on a variety of dental hygiene services on a sample day with eight 1-hour appointments.

The results for the day show revenue of $1,085. As a student, this kind of day appears overwhelming, especially since many have had three- to four-hour clinic sessions during their programs. However, as dental hygienists enter the working environment, this may be a schedule that they find within the first 30 days of employment.

TABLE 8-2 Sample Daily Schedule

Dentist Room 1		Dentist Room 2		Dentist Room 3		RDH	
8:00	($650)	Single X-ray	($45)			8:00	($175)
Single crown		Check tooth				1 quadrant root plane	
		9:00	($220)	9:30	($165)	9:30	($70)
		2 composite fillings		New patient exam and full set of X-rays		Adult prophy	
10:30	($450)					10:30	($70)
Root canal—molar						Adult prophy	
						11:30	($120)
						4 sealants	
Lunch	12:00	Lunch		Lunch		Lunch	

TABLE 8-3 Sample of Dental Hygiene Production

Quantity	Procedure	Fee	Production
5	Adult prophylaxis treatments	$75	$375
2	Root planing/quadrants	200	400
1	Child prophylaxis treatment with fluoride	65	65
4	Bitewing radiographs	75	300
1	Full set of radiographs	110	110
4	Sealants	30	120
		Total	**$1,370**

The cost of doing dental hygiene business is equally important to discuss here. However, the costs of utilities, such as electricity, water, and gas, are not discussed here because this model uses the dental hygienist as an employee within a practice. Utilities would be used by the employer also and would be used in calculating overhead for the practice as a whole. For dental hygienists who seek or enter independent practice, utilities would need to be included and also calculated in total costs. So how does overhead affect dental hygiene? Mainly, it has to do with the oral hygiene aids given to each patient and with the salary of the dental hygienist. If the dental hygienist receives benefits, this too would be an expense for the employer.

The sample day given in Table 8-2 itemizes approximate daily expenses. Profit for dental hygiene procedures will not be as large as dental procedures (Table 8-3). The cost for a quadrant of root planing is far from the cost of a crown or three-unit bridge. In addition, this sample does not take into account patients who cancel or fail to make their appointment at the last minute. It also does not take into account insurance payments received. Thus, profit will fluctuate on a daily basis. What may not fluctuate is the salary and benefit package paid to the dental hygienist, unless the compensation is based on a percentage of production (to be explained in Chapter 10). Although there are numerous factors that are seen daily in the dental practice, a profit is likely to be realized.

Creating Daily Schedules

Those with previous experience understand that the practice as a whole must create a schedule that is productive for the business yet workable for the staff. For new dental hygienists entering the dental business, an understanding of how the daily schedule must flow will be essential to both the financial bottom line and the smooth transition from patient to patient for the dentist and the assistants. What is considered when creating the dental office work schedule? First, there will be the dentists' schedule, then the dental hygienists' schedule. The only time they may cross paths will be when the dentist must perform a periodic examination for the dental hygiene patient or evaluate other concerns. Remember that this is generally discussed during the huddles each morning.

The dentist's schedule will consist of a variety of restorative procedures that are placed at specific times throughout the day. For example, perhaps the dentist prefers long procedures, such as fixed bridges, crowns, or root canals, first thing in the morning or immediately following the lunch hour. Then other procedures that take less time, such as smaller restorations, examinations, or extractions, are allocated around the more extensive procedures. The dentist will provide dental hygiene exams at stopping points within the procedures that are on his or her schedule.

TABLE 8-4 Sample Approximate Daily Expenses for a Dental Hygiene Day		
	Oral Health Aids and Procedures	**Cost to Practice**
8 patients =	8 toothbrushes @ $2.00	$16.00
	8 floss dispensers @ $.25	$2.00
	2 interdental brushes @ $1.00	$2.00
	8 toothpaste tubes @ $1.00	$8.00
	Total	**$28.00**
If radiographs are included:		
	4 BWX @ $2.00	$8.00
	1 FMX @ $9.00	$9.00
Sealant material	4 @ $1.00	$4.00
	Total	**$21.00**
DH salary	$32.00/hour × 8	$256.00
Benefits (if applicable @ 10% of salary)		$25.60
Total expenses for the day		**$330.60**
Profit received by the practice $1,370−330.60		**$1,039.40**

As the schedule is designed by the allocation of specific procedures, the business also has financial goals that may be established each month during staff meetings or on an annual basis. For example, perhaps the monthly production goal for the practice as a whole is $50,000. This figure then dictates the daily goal, which is now $1,729 (for a 28-day month). Taking the daily goal, the dentist will focus on procedures that can assist in meeting the financial goal, and so too will the dental hygienist's schedule be designed to help meet the daily and monthly goals. Table 8-4 provides an example of how a daily schedule may be designed to meet the financial goals.

As depicted in the morning sample schedule, the dentist has procedures that will create $1,530 in production, and the dental hygienist has $435 in production for a total of $1,965. This already exceeds the established goal set by the practice. Thus, it is not a difficult task to reach the production goals that the staff or dentist chooses to set for themselves in order to be financially successful. When a dental practice works with management or business consultants, the staff often participates in setting production goals to ensure that patients are well cared for and that the staff is not rushing around trying to stay on time with the schedule.

DENTAL INSURANCE AND HYGIENE SERVICES

Fees for dental hygiene services vary throughout the country. In addition, dental insurance coverage varies greatly, depending on the type of insurance consumers carry, and many consumers have no dental insurance coverage. Payment for dental and dental hygiene services will also vary, anywhere from zero to 100%. Insurance companies will also vary their payment depending on the type of hygiene services provided to the consumer. For example, a regular prophylaxis may be covered and paid at 100%, whereas quadrant root planing may be covered and paid at 50% to 70%. Again, it depends on what type of dental coverage the consumer holds.

Common Insurance Plans

Although there are a number of insurance plans available to the consumer, those described here are among the most common found in dental practices, both private and public.

PRIVATE-PAY PLANS Private-pay patients are those who do not have insurance and will pay for services rendered out-of-pocket. These patients will pay the **usual, customary, and reasonable** (UCR) fees that have been determined by the dentist owner of the practice. Most dental corporations use UCR fees. Such fees can be found in all privately owned dental practices and typically will be submitted for approval to insurance companies that assist in maintaining the level of fees in a particular geographic area. For example, if Practice A charges $70 per dental prophylaxis, Practice B may not be able to charge $90 for the same service if located in the same city or county. Thus, the consumer benefits from this type of regulation and will not feel overcharged for the same basic service. Insurance carriers paying the practice from UCR fees generally pay by percentage. For example, if the prophylaxis fee is $70, the insurance payment may be 70%, and then the patient must pay 30%.

PREFERRED PROVIDER ORGANIZATION (PPO) The amount of payment to the practice or dentist is set in a fee schedule determined by the insurance company. When the dentist bills for services, payment will not exceed the agreed-on fee schedule. In addition, patients generally have a copayment for each visit and procedure that will be set and limited by the **PPO** plan. This helps keep out-of-pocket expenses lower for the consumer.

HMOS AND DHMOS **Health maintenance organizations** (HMOs) and **dental health maintenance organizations** (DHMOs) are other types of insurance carriers that may limit dental care to within the organization, including their own dental facilities. The HMOs have accepted responsibility and financial risks for providing dental services. Both HMOs and DHMOs may also be limited to providing coverage to consumers within a specific geographic area, such as a limited number of ZIP codes or counties. Payments to the dentists again tend to be based on a specific scale or percentage based on UCR fees but determined by the insurance carrier or HMO corporation rather than the dentist.

STATE-ASSISTED HEALTH PLANS **State assistance** for medical and dental coverage is another way for low-income families (especially children) to receive needed oral health care. Each state has guidelines and qualifications, and there may be a limited number of dental practices offering to accept this kind of dental coverage into their practice. Generally, reimbursement rates to the dentist in a state-assisted health plan are far below UCR fees and thus often do not cover the cost to provide services. Therefore, in many communities, there may be few private practices offering to accept state-assisted families. Some communities will provide community health and dental facilities to those receiving state aid. Students may become familiar with these families or these facilities during their community oral health course, and PPO, HMO, and DHMO coverage are major factors for managed care.

CAPITATION SYSTEMS **Capitation** *systems* are based on the fact that the dentist, not an insurance company, takes the risk for delivering dental care. The dentist is compensated a fixed fee based on the number of patients enrolled in this system rather than on the type of services rendered. For example, if 100 people are enrolled in a dental capitation plan, the dentist may be compensated $10 for each person enrolled regardless of whether they are actually patients in the practice.

Then, for treatment provided to those enrolled, the office will bill the carrier for services rendered. These are only a few ways for a new practice to realize early revenue. Incorporating these types of clientele in a dental practice requires business savvy and advanced scheduling skills for the practice to realize an acceptable profit.

Insurance Billing Procedures

The type of insurance held will determine billing procedures for patients with insurance coverage. Some insurance companies may require their own dental billing form. Others may accept a universal form that can be used for numerous insurance companies. State plans may have a specific form designed to meet their specific needs.

PREAUTHORIZATION   **Preauthorization** of planned treatment may be required by insurance companies or requested by the patient. This means that once the dental hygienist has determined how to approach a patient's treatment, the insurance company may require prior authorization. For example, if the patient has been determined to need quadrant therapy in order to return to better oral health, the insurance company may request a copy of the radiographs and periodontal assessment to confirm that quadrant therapy is warranted. For the insurance company, this is a way to monitor the expenses paid for services and to monitor the treatment received by the patient. Additionally, most insurance companies will place a limit on how often procedures can be performed. For example, periodontal treatment may be allowed only once every three years. There are insurance companies and dental coverage that do not require preauthorization for treatment. Each insurance plan, much like each patient, will need to be viewed independently.

Insurance Codes

As the oral health provider, the dental hygienist will want to be familiar with the insurance processes that are required from the practice. Those who are familiar with dental insurance have worked with dental insurance billing codes and use them to help design appropriate treatment plans for their patients. Current Dental Terminology (CDT) is a coding system published by the American Dental Association. All dental procedures are given a specific code number, placed in categories such as preventive, diagnostic, or periodontics, and are used when billing insurance companies. Using CDT codes make the billing process more accurate, providing a timely reimbursement to the practice. Table 8-5 gives examples of some of the insurance codes that are pertinent to dental hygiene treatment. It will be an advantage for the dental hygienist to become familiar with these codes so that patient treatment and insurance coverage are maximized.

Excluded Treatments

Although Table 8-5 represents only a portion of insurance codes that are used in the dental office, this will help the dental hygienist understand what is available when planning treatment. It should be mentioned at this point that although many patients may have some insurance benefits, not all procedures may be included in their particular plan. For example, notice the code D1310, nutritional counseling. Even though this code is included in all UCR fees and recognized by dental insurance companies, many plans do not pay benefits for patients to receive this treatment. Therefore, it is wise to review what may or may not be covered in the patient's insurance plan

TABLE 8-5 **(2009–10) Insurance Codes and Nomenclature for Dental Hygiene–Related Procedures Abbreviated**

D0100-0999 I. Diagnostic

Clinical and oral evaluation

D0120 Periodic oral evaluation—established patient

D0140 Limited oral evaluation—problem focused

D0150 Comprehensive oral evaluation—new or established patient

D0160 Detailed and extensive oral evaluation—problem focused, by report

D0180 Comprehensive periodontal evaluation—new or established patient

Radiographs

D0210 Intraoral—complete series (including bitewings)

D0220 Intraoral—periapical; first film

D0230 Intraoral—periapical; each additional film

D0240 Intraoral—occlusal film

D0270 Bitewings—single film

D0272 Bitewings—two films

D0274 Bitewings—four films

D0330 Panoramic film

Tests and laboratory examinations

D0415 Collection of microorganisms for culture and sensitivity

D0417 Collection and preparation of saliva sample for laboratory diagnostic testing

D0418 Analysis of saliva sample

D0421 Genetic test for susceptibility to oral diseases

D0425 Caries susceptibility tests

D0431 Adjunctive prediagnostic test that aids in detection of mucosal abnormalities including premalignant and malignant lesions, not to include cytology or biopsy procedures

D0460 Pulp vitality tests

D0470 Diagnostic casts

D0502 Other oral pathology procedures, by report

D0999 Unspecified diagnostic procedure, by report

D 1000–1999 II. Preventive

Dental prophylaxis

D1110 Prophylaxis—adult

D1120 Prophylaxis—child

D1203 Topical application of fluoride—child

D1204 Topical application of fluoride—adult

D1206 Topical fluoride varnish; therapeutic application for moderate to high caries risk patients

D1310 Nutritional counseling for the control of dental disease

D1320 Tobacco counseling for the control and prevention of oral disease

D1330 Oral hygiene instructions

D1351 Sealant—per tooth

TABLE 8-5 *(Continued)*

D4000–4999 V. Periodontics

Adjunctive periodontal surgery

D4341 Periodontal scaling and root planing—4 or more teeth per quadrant

D4355 Full mouth debridement to enable comprehensive periodontal evaluation and diagnosis

D4381 Localized delivery of chemotherapeutic agents via controlled release vehicle into diseased crevicular tissue, per tooth, by report

D4910 Periodontal maintenance

D4920 Unscheduled dressing change (by someone other than the treating dentist)

D4999 Unspecified periodontal procedure, by report

Miscellaneous services

D9910 Application of desensitizing medicament

D9920 Behavior management, by report

D9999 Unspecified adjunctive procedure, by report

---

with the office manager or insurance coordinator, as that person may have a better understanding of how the insurance company handles these types of services.

How various insurance and managed care plans affect the overall income and profitability of the practice is an area too extensive for the scope of this text. For those who seek positions in facilities that accept many of these programs, expanded information will be readily available to assist in the comprehension of how these programs operate on a daily basis.

Case Study Follow-up #3

After reading about the complexities of insurance plans and how it may affect dental hygiene treatment, what kind of role can you play, as a leader in your office that will benefit both patients and the practice?

CONTINUING CARE AND RECARE SYSTEMS

During any dental hygiene education, students become familiar with continuing care or recare (formerly recall) systems. To assist patients in maintaining oral health, the dental hygienist wants to see them periodically. This means that the patient is recalled for continuing care at certain intervals.

Continuing Care Systems

A continuing care system is integral to continued patient flow in the practice and can be seen as the lifeline to long-term success. Although most often patients will receive an oral prophylaxis and examination, many will also be seen for various other reasons, some of which apply to post-dental treatment: extractions, orthodontic treatment, and follow-up visits after endodontic therapy.

Extensive research and knowledge of the cause and effect of periodontal health and its effect on systemic health recognizes that patient education is more important than ever if the dental hygienist and the patient are to be successful in oral health care. Successful systems will incorporate several factors: oral health education, motivation, consistent follow-up, and appropriate treatment. Continuing care systems are varied, and each practice will use the system that best suits its needs for managing patients.

ADVANCED APPOINTMENT SYSTEMS   The **advanced appointment system** is increasingly becoming the most widely used in many areas. As each patient completes a dental hygiene visit, he or she is scheduled for the next visit prior to leaving the office. By scheduling in advance, the patient has committed that day and time to the dental hygienist. The disadvantages are that many patients do not know their work or personal schedules that far in advance. Additionally, the dentist and the dental hygienist cannot predict that they will not be ill on the day the patient has scheduled.

MAIL SYSTEM OPTIONS   A **mail system** consists of mailing a card to the patients during the month they are due for their regular appointment. This places the responsibility on the patient, as he or she will need to call and schedule the appointment. The disadvantage is that the patient may forget to call or may ignore the notice. With many computer systems and software programs, most practices enter recare due dates as the patient is dismissed. Later, a report can be printed showing the last date of service, the type of service received, the specific interval recommended by the dental hygienist, and the date of the patient's next appointment.

ELECTRONIC OPTIONS   Today, more people are using e-mail, social networks, and text messaging to communicate and accomplish daily tasks. With Internet communication as an option, patients may prefer to have the office contact them via e-mail or text messaging to smartphones.

Continuing Care Objectives

In creating an effective hygiene department, the dental hygienist can identify objectives that the continuing care system should address. These objectives could include the following:

- Customizing the approach to treatment
- Encouraging patient compliance and return for future appointments
- Obtaining a commitment from the patient to accept treatment recommendations
- Motivating patients to take an active role in their oral health and treatment
- Educating patients on the significance of continuing care and its value relative to restorative treatment

In addition to establishing workable and attainable objectives, the dental hygiene department may decide to incorporate a philosophy that all participants can apply to their everyday working routine. It is imperative for each practitioner in the department to establish and document the diagnosis as it pertains to the patient's current oral health condition. Each patient should be informed of the diagnosis and counseled as to the recommended treatment and any options that apply. Finally, treatment will be provided by the professional as indicated by the diagnosis and discussed with the patient.

Developing an effective hygiene department may be a challenge for those who are asked to participate. Many factors need to be considered. Therefore, planning plays a significant role during initiation stages. Continuous review of the philosophy and objectives will be required by all participants to best maintain smooth operations.

TIME MANAGEMENT

For a new graduate, time management is the most common concern. Most programs may have allowed students three to four hours for each clinic session. Now, on the first day of a new job, the dental hygienist has been cut down to one hour for each patient. Additionally, he or she is expected to see an average of eight patients that day and to stay on schedule. After all, the patients are not new to the practice. They anticipate the same appointment they usually attend at each recall visit. You, as the new employee and new dental hygienist, are the newest addition to the practice.

VARYING POLICIES   Many practices allow the dental hygienist 60-minute appointments. However, this is not always the case. Some offices allow 45- or 50-minute appointments. The procedures performed by the clinician will be identical regardless of what time allowance is given per appointment. As a result, the new practitioner must plan the hour or time allotted in such a manner that all patients can be seen on time. Time management is an issue that many employers are aware of, and many are willing to work with you as you gain experience in the office. One of the dental assistants may be assigned to the dental hygienist as he or she becomes familiar with the equipment, location of materials, and schedule. Thus, do not hesitate to discuss this aspect of the new position during interviews.

How can time management be addressed when beginning a new position? One area to consider is radiographs. Discuss the possibility of having one of the dental assistants take radiographs that may be required for those scheduled with the dental hygienist. This will allow extra time in that hour for clinical needs, such as periodontal charting or scaling. Other suggestions may arise during discussion of time management with potential employers.

LIMITED TIME CONSTRAINTS   For those who obtain employment in practices that accept PPO, HMO, or state assistance plans, the time allotment for dental hygiene appointments could be much shorter. Recall that managed care programs require special scheduling in order for the practice to break even or realize a profit. This leads to 45- and sometimes even 30-minute appointments. If you decide to work in a practice that appoints patients at 30-minute intervals, it is highly recommended to have an assigned dental assistant. This helps to maintain higher quality care and patient education.

Again, the dental hygienist is expected to provide normal hygiene services regardless of the time allowed. Many new practitioners are unable to work within these time constraints. Most often, the new practitioner has difficulty feeling as though he or she is benefiting the patient. This can result in ethical dilemmas or distress. Ethical obligations for dental hygienists for patients are at the forefront of every procedure performed. Thus, when interviewing for dental hygiene positions that include managed care programs, be sure to discuss the time allowed for procedures and be sure that you are ethically and morally comfortable that the patient is receiving the best care available.

Time management will improve quickly for each new practitioner. Open communication with the dental assistant and employer will assist in making the transition smoother while increasing efficiency with each appointment.

WORKING WITH OTHER DENTAL HYGIENISTS

When entering a new position, be sure to ask the same questions as for any interview. During dental hygiene school, most students purchase their own instruments. When working in one or more practice, the employer may supply the instruments; however, more than one clinician will be sharing the same sets. This may become problematic since each clinician sharpens and scales differently. Several options can be employed to alleviate problems with instruments when shared. The employer may decide to purchase instruments for each hygienist; thus, each will have several sets to last an entire day. Another option is for the dental hygienist to purchase his or her own instruments. If the dental hygienist is employed in one office, the instruments can be stored in the operatory. If employed in two or more offices, the dental hygienist may choose to travel with his or her instruments.

Some practices provide the dental hygienist with a dental assistant. This may be a rare convenience for many seasoned practitioners, yet there are practices that incorporate this aspect. Sometimes the employer provides a dental assistant only during the transition period of the new association with the practice. Dental assistants assigned to the dental hygienists will perform adjunct duties, such as taking radiographs, setting up instrument trays, sterilization procedures, seating patients, and numerous other activities. This arrangement will allow for increased production by the hygiene department, less stress among the clinicians, and efficient appointments for the patients.

WORKING AS A PUBLIC HEALTH DENTAL HYGIENIST

Another area for those entering a dental hygiene career is the public health arena. There are multifaceted ways the dental hygienist can improve oral health through public organizations. Many public health agencies, whether at the local, state, or national level, have a need for health care experts on advisory committees, task forces, or boards. A dental hygienist employed in public health can design oral health programs that will target specific groups in their community or state. They can also participate in needs assessment data collection so that public health funds and programs can be designed and implemented to meet such needs. Additionally, there are groups that may require oral health education, and often the dental hygienist will be called to provide such presentations.

Working as a public health dental hygienist will often require increased organizational and business skills. Funding and budgetary concerns often are an issue in the design and administration of oral health programs or projects. The dental hygienist can be the ideal administrator because of his or her extensive oral health education and can use such knowledge to improve oral health at all levels of need in any community. When employed in a private practice, the clinician focuses on the needs of each consumer as an individual. The public health dental hygienist employs much of the same skills to a much larger degree and can spend more time on evaluation of how well dental programs succeed.

There are many dental hygienists who work full time in private practice, yet also participate in small ways assisting with public oral health projects. Each health care professional has the skill and opportunity to contribute to many public health organizations, yet these opportunities are often overlooked. Since the dental hygiene profession has such diversity in career options, new graduates are encouraged to explore the many options available to them in their community as well as around the world.

CAREER ALTERNATIVES

Throughout a dental hygienist's education, students are likely exposed to many other practitioners who hold careers in other areas of the profession. For example, students may have had a corporate representative present a seminar on dental hygiene products or how to work with products when in private practice. A career in dental hygiene is not limited to clinical practice. Many graduates are likely to begin their careers working with a private office in order to gain higher clinical skill and patient assessment techniques. The interaction with and shared knowledge of colleagues in this environment are essential to the overall knowledge of clinical dental hygiene practice. Once employed in the private sector for a while, clinicians may begin to search for other opportunities to broaden their careers.

Six Roles of the Dental Hygienist

The six roles of the dental hygienist include:

- administrator
- clinician
- change agent
- researcher
- educator
- consumer advocate

Dental hygienists are encouraged to keep these roles in mind as they continue in their careers yet find that their interest in dental hygiene shifts toward another aspect of the profession.

ADMINISTRATOR   The role of administrator may include working with private or government agencies, such as health departments, special oral health task forces, and college education programs. Many agencies will seek the expertise of an oral health professional when setting goals for improved health in any community.

CLINICIAN   Dental hygienists are most often employed as clinicians in a private practice setting working as a member of the dental team. Their most important role is oral health education and providing dental hygiene services in partnership with their patients maintaining optimal oral health.

CHANGE AGENT   Change agents are those who seek to work with legislators, lobbyists, or both to protect and augment the scope of dental hygiene practice. Many dental hygienists active in their professional associations work as change agents, establishing new legislation for their states.

RESEARCHER   Dental hygienists may change direction at sometime in their career and go into research. This may include working with one of many corporate dental entities to develop and test new products for oral health.

EDUCATOR   The field of education is experiencing a lack of students interested in teaching dental education, whether in dental hygiene or in dentistry. Many dental hygiene programs continuously seek qualified applicants to increase their faculty. Higher education will be required to fill teaching positions, and those interested in a career in education are encouraged to seek a baccalaureate degree at minimum, yet many educational institutions prefer a master's or a doctoral degree.

CONSUMER ADVOCATE   Consumer advocates may also include change agents, and/or they may work at the community level with private organizations, such as long-term care facilities, creating oral health programs that target special groups. They will also focus on legislation that will help protect the oral health of consumers.

ADDITIONAL RESPONSIBILITIES   Another aspect of dental hygiene practice is the expansion of practice to include limited restorative procedures. Several states, such as Delaware, Florida, and Washington, allow dental hygienists to place and finish composite restorations, place and remove temporary fillings and crowns, along with placing bases and liners (ADA 2007 Survey of Legal Provisions for Delegating Intraoral Functions to Dental Assistants and Dental Hygienists, 2007). Adding this array of duties to the scope of practice for dental hygiene enhances the practitioner to expand their working venues. This also serves to address the needs of communities that may have limited access to traditional dental practices.

Forensics has become a career path for both dentists and dental hygienists since the unfortunate events of September 11, the airline crash in the Florida Everglades, and others. Often it involves reviewing radiographs and taking alginate impressions to determine identification of human remains, and dental professionals are increasingly sought.

As mentioned, many practitioners may be content to work in the private sector for a while and then move on to another aspect of the dental hygiene field. It will be necessary to seek and obtain higher education for many of these career alternatives.

LIFELONG LEARNING

In most states, part of being a licensed health care provider means continuing one's education to maintain an active license status. Most states require that licensed dental hygienists attend continuing education courses that focus on patient care. Each state differs in the number of hours required per license cycle. For example, to maintain a California license, dental hygienists are required to attend 25 hours of continuing education courses within two years, as their license must be renewed every 2 years.

Because the dental hygienist is providing patient care, it will be necessary to stay abreast of instrument or treatment techniques, medications, systemic conditions, and trends in oral health, as this benefits the patient. Once having graduated from a dental hygiene program, many believe that their "school days" are over. However, it will be imperative to attend continuing education courses to maintain high-quality care throughout the course of any oral health care career.

Summary

The dental hygiene diagnosis, or process of care, is separate from the dental diagnosis. Analysis of factual information provided by patients and determining the human deficit present are required for the dental hygienist to develop the appropriate diagnosis for patients' current oral health conditions. Additionally, the dental hygienist must deal with the beliefs, attitudes, and perceptions of his

or her patients, and this will require effective communication skills to ensure patient compliance.

Take care to focus on healthy areas of the mouth as well problem areas. Some patients complain that the dental hygienist reprimands them. Turning the approach toward the positive will allow the dental hygienist to use the strengths of his or her patients rather than point out the weaknesses.

Patients want to be recognized for their accomplishments; thus, refocusing on their achievements may prove beneficial in maintaining patient compliance.

When employed in private practice, each practitioner has the opportunity to use experts and specialists associated with the employer and the practice. Dental hygienists also have the opportunity to work with HMOs as well as community facilities that are focused on oral health services.

Maximizing your skills as a professional dental hygienist includes understanding your total background as well as acquired information learned on a daily basis. Formal education, continuing education as a lifelong learner, and education from interactions with employers, coworkers, and patients contribute to your professional composition. Everyone benefits when these skills are used to their greatest potential.

Critical Thinking

1. Describe the differences between the dental diagnosis and the dental hygiene diagnosis. How does the dental hygiene diagnosis influence treatment planning and insurance coverage?

2. Develop several scenarios for a dental hygiene schedule and calculate production and expenses. What is the resulting profit for the practice?

3. Using Table 8-5, identify the insurance codes that would be used for four quadrants of root planing, a full set of radiographs, and a periodontal maintenance visit.

4. Given 1 hour for a dental hygiene visit, list the procedures to be performed on a patient who has come in for a 6-month prophylaxis. What would be the standard of care in this case? The procedures should also include periodontal charting, radiographs, and an examination by the dentist. Using this list, determine how much time will be needed for each procedure in order to stay within the 60-minute time period.

   a. What would be the time needed for the same procedures given a 45-minute appointment?

   b. How about a 30-minute appointment? Can you identify areas that will suffer when the time becomes too short?

5. Take 5 minutes and list leadership traits you feel you hold. Pair with a classmate and identify leadership traits of your classmate. Compare and discuss the traits on your list.

6. Contact your local health department for information on current public health programs that may be ongoing in your community.

CHAPTER 9

Alternate Practice Models

Future Trends for Oral Health Care

OBJECTIVES

After reading the material in this chapter, you will be able to

- Describe different models for alternate practice.
- Discuss legislative barriers to alternate practice.
- List different duties for dental hygienists in alternative practice and dental therapists.
- Develop a business plan for an alternative practice model.

KEY TERMS

Dental therapist
  (DT, ADT)
Mid-level oral health
  provider

Registered dental hygienist
  in alternative practice
  (RDHAP)
Alternative practice

Collaborative practice
Independent practice
Unsupervised practice

INTRODUCTION

Many, if not the majority of graduates will find themselves in a private practice setting. The majority of dentists choose to own and operate their own practice, whether in general dentistry or in one of the dental specialties. However, dental hygiene services are needed in other settings and a need to increase access to dental care continues. Generally, under the laws of most states, dental hygienists can work in elementary school settings, nonprofit community dental facilities, hospitals, military bases, and federal Native American reservations under the appropriate supervision. This allows oral health care workers the opportunity to increase access to care for all individuals.

In 2000, the *U.S. Surgeon General's Report* addressed the oral health of America for the first time (U.S. Department of Health and Human Services, 2000). This report brought forward the reality of access to care needed by millions, many of whom are children. Organized dentistry, dental hygiene, and many other health organizations are working to make improvements in this area. As a result, new workforce models are being developed that will allow dental hygienists and others to target rural areas around the country and provide much-needed basic dental care and education. This chapter describes the movement of dental hygiene toward **alternative practice** settings and new oral health workforce models currently established in many nations of the world along with new programs offered in the United States. This change in course for dentistry and dental hygiene has faced numerous challenges, yet it now gains more acceptance and promotion in order to decrease oral health disparities.

Case Study

California has two dental hygiene schools offering the **Registered Dental Hygienist in Alternative Practice (RDHAP)** program. The University of the Pacific (UOP) in San Francisco provides an online format, whereas West Los Angeles Community College (WLAC) offers the course through traditional classroom instruction. Additionally, Normandale Community College in Minnesota and the University of Minnesota Dental School now offer bachelor and master degree programs for the **dental therapist**.

As you read this chapter consider, the following: Locate the websites of each college or university offering the alternate dental or dental hygiene degrees. Then locate a geographic area in your state, or within neighboring states that have an unmet need for oral health because of a lack of providers, or due to access to care issues. Once you decide on your target population, select a practice model (dental therapist, RDHAP, or collaborative practice) and create a business plan that will allow you to operate in an alternative setting. Use the business plan template found in MyHealthProfessionsKit, along with some of the Internet resources. Assume you have completed an alternate dental hygiene or dental therapist program and are now licensed in the state you are going to practice. You may also have to assume that the state dental practice act allows alternate practice.

OVERVIEW OF ALTERNATIVE PRACTICE IN THE UNITED STATES

Independent practice made its first appearance as early as 1976. Linda Krol, a California dental hygienist, was the first to own and manage her own practice. This innovative thinking caused organized dentistry to look closer at who could own a practice and the scope of practice for dental hygienists. So began the movement toward expanded functions for auxiliaries.

In 1986, California began its Health Manpower Pilot Project (HMPP #139) designed to study the safety of, and access to, dental hygiene services in unsupervised settings. Approximately twenty dental hygienists participated in the pilot project providing dental hygiene services to the public. This project went on for ten years without legal incident, proving that services could be safely provided with little or no supervision of a dentist. Legal success was realized in 1998 with the licensure for the registered dental hygienist in alternative practice. Today, there are over 300 dental hygienists who own and operate their own dental hygiene business in California. Some are freestanding offices, while others choose to use mobile equipment and provide services in nursing care or residential care facilities.

As delivery of oral health care seeks progressive and innovative licensure, many states find themselves with more dental hygienists obtaining advanced education and licensure for some version of alternative practice. Colorado successfully passed legislation in 1986 allowing independent or **unsupervised practice** for dental hygienists. They could also own their practice and purchase equipment conducive to providing dental hygiene services. In 1999, New Mexico dental hygienists began practicing in what is termed a **collaborative practice** based on criteria that have been established by a committee and state governing board. This includes allowing the dental hygienist to provide education, assessment, preventive, therapeutic, and clinical services without supervision. They, too, can work in a variety of settings: schools, nursing facilities, and private dental hygiene practice. At present, 19 states have some form of alternate scope of practice based on changes in law, supervision, and access to care needs as shown in Table 9-1. This is one part of the movement toward a future pathway for the dental hygienist as a professional.

TABLE 9-1   Allowable Duties, Settings, and Supervision for Dental Hygienists by State

Alaska 2008	Can provide the entire scope of dental hygiene practice along with other duties as specified by a collaborative agreement; dentist does not have to diagnose or be present.
Arizona 2004	Any dental hygiene services specified in the affiliated practice agreement except root planing, local anesthesia, nitrous oxide, or placing sutures can be done unsupervised.
California 1998	Dental hygienists endorsed as RDHAPs (registered dental hygienist in alternative practice) may provide services without supervision for homebound persons or at schools, residential facilities, institutions, and in dental health professional shortage areas for up to 18 months, and provide further services if the patient obtains a prescription from a dentist or physician. RDHAPs may own an alternative dental hygiene practice.
Colorado 1987	Services include dental hygiene diagnosis, X-rays, remove deposits, accretions, and stains, curettage without anesthesia, apply fluorides and other recognized preventive agents, oral inspection and charting, and topical anesthetic; local anesthesia requires general supervision; all other services do not require supervision.
Connecticut 1999	Services are provided in school settings, institutions, group homes, and public health settings; oral prophylaxis, removal of deposits, accretions, and stains, root planning, sealants, assessment, and treatment planning can all be done unsupervised.
Idaho 2004	Services are provided in hospitals, long-term care facilities, public, and migrant health facilities; services must be authorized by the dentist.
Iowa 2004	All dental hygiene services (except local anesthesia and nitrous) may be provided once to each patient; to perform repeat services other than assessment, screening and fluoride, dentist must examine; settings are mainly public health and institutions.
Kansas 2003	Services are provided in public health, school, and institutional settings; hygienists can provide prophylaxis, application of fluoride, dental hygiene instruction; hygienists must have a sponsoring agreement with a dentist.
Maine 2008	Dental hygienists can practice independently, without supervision under any setting; they can provide the entire scope of practice; they must follow manufacturers' recommendations on all products used; they must provide patients with a referral plan for any services requiring a dentist.
Massachusetts 2009	Full scope of practice and procedures authorized by the board as a delegable procedure for dental hygienists in private practice under general supervision; all public health settings.

TABLE 9-1   (Continued)

Michigan 2005	Dental hygienists can be recognized as a special grantee and work on patients who are not assigned to a dentist; dental hygiene services are provided under general supervision.
Minnesota 2001, 2009	Dental hygienists can be employed in health care facility or program and see patients before they see a dentist; they must have a collaborative agreement with a dentist; all dental hygiene services can be provided; state laws passed to provide education and scope of practice for dental therapists and alternate oral health care providers.
Missouri 2001	Limited services including oral prophylaxis, sealants, and fluorides are done in public health settings.
Montana 2003	Dental hygienists must obtain a limited license for public health settings; services include prophylaxis, fluoride, root planning, sealants, polish restorations, X-rays for diagnosis by a dentists, and oral cancer screening.
Nebraska 2007	The Department of Health may authorize a dental hygienist to provide preventive treatment to children unsupervised.
New Hampshire 1993	Instruction in oral hygiene, topical fluorides, oral prophylaxis, assess medical/ dental history, periodontal probing, charting, sealants, public health supervision is required, and settings include hospitals, institutions, and homebound.
New Mexico 1999	Collaborative practice agreements must be in place; standing orders include services for preliminary assessment, X-rays, oral prophylaxis and fluoride treatment without prior authorization; case-by-case authorization required in some procedures (such as sealants and root planing).
New York 2006	A dental hygienist can work in any setting (private or public) and perform dental hygiene duties; the dentist must be available for diagnosis, consultation, and evaluation.
Nevada 1998	Dental hygienists may obtain a public health endorsement to work as public health dental health hygienists in schools, community centers, hospitals, and nursing homes without supervision.
Oklahoma 2003	The dentist may authorize a dental hygienist to perform services one time outside of the dental office setting prior to the dental examination.
Oregon 1997	All dental hygiene services, except some (local anesthesia, pit and fissure sealants, denture relines, temporary restorations, radiographs, and nitrous oxide) must be supervised by a dentist; dental hygienists may prescribe fluorides and assess the need for sealants; the dental hygienist must have a limited access permit (LAP).
Pennsylvania 2007	Dental hygienists can practice as public health dental hygiene practitioners providing a variety of services in any public health settings.
Rhode Island 2006	Under general supervision, dental hygienists can provide services in nursing facilities.
South Carolina 2003	Under general supervision, a prophylaxis, fluoride, and sealants can be performed if the dental hygienist is contacted or employed by the Department of Health and Environmental Control.
Texas 2001	The dentist can authorize dental hygienists to provide the entire scope of dental hygiene services for a period of 6 months without a dentist seeing the patient first; the patient must be referred to the dentist and the dental hygienist may not perform a second set of services unless the patient has had a dental examination.

(continued)

TABLE 9-1	**Allowable Duties, Settings, and Supervision for Dental Hygienists by State** (*Continued*)
Vermont 2008	Under general supervision agreement, the dental hygienist can provide services in public health settings.
Virginia 2009 Pilot Project	The Virginia Pilot Project seeks to assess the impact dental hygienists practicing in an expanded capacity under remote supervision have on increasing access to dental health care for underserved populations; hygienists can provide initial examination of teeth and surrounding areas, prophylaxis, scaling, sealants, topical fluoride, education services, assessment, and screening.
Washington 1984	Dental hygienist can practice unsupervised in public health facilities, nursing homes, hospitals, and institutions.
West Virginia 2008	Unsupervised practice is allowed for dental hygienists meeting specific qualifications; all settings are public health in nature: group homes, hospitals, schools, and nursing facilities.
Wisconsin 2007	New statute 447.06 does not require the presence or supervision of a dentist in a public or private school, a dental or dental hygiene school or a facility owned by a local health department.

Adapted from: *Direct Access States*, American Dental Hygienists' Association (2010).

Information presented in Table 9-1 shows not only the settings and supervision for dental hygienists as they work to address oral health issues in their state, it also shows the first year in which state laws were passed making significant changes. Getting legislative approval can take many years and the expertise of lobbyists working with each state's dental hygiene association. Many of these states have gone on to pass or modify more laws regarding scope of practice and supervision. By doing so, dental hygienists are gaining more ground in addressing access to care barriers and the ability to practice independently.

Case Study Follow-up #1

Using either the information in Table 1, or your state's dental practice act, research the scope of practice for dental hygiene in your state. Does it allow for alternate practice settings? Are there limitations? If so, what are they?

ALTERNATE PRACTICE MODELS

International Models for the Dental Therapist

NEW ZEALAND   Today there are over 600 dental therapists in New Zealand. However, this concept began in 1921 under the name of dental nurses. The origin of dental therapy is attributed to Britain and New Zealand in the early 1900s and targeted children ages 6 to 14. Dental therapists are still mainly assigned to schools and provide services for children. Education programs for dental therapists are three years in length culminating in a bachelor's degree in oral health science from the University of Otaga or Auckland, or a diploma in dental therapy from a New Zealand educational institution or a certificate in dental therapy issued by the

BOX 9-1

A Brief List of Duties for Dental Therapists in New Zealand

The scope of practice includes

- obtaining medical histories and consulting with other health practitioners as appropriate
- examination of oral tissues, diagnosis of dental caries and recognition of abnormalities
- preparation of an oral care plan
- informed consent procedures
- administration of local anesthetic using dentoalveolar infiltration, inferior dental nerve block and topical local anesthetic techniques
- preparation of cavities and restoration of primary and permanent teeth using direct placement of appropriate dental materials
- extraction of primary teeth
- pulp capping in primary and permanent teeth
- preventive dentistry including cleaning, polishing and scaling (to remove deposits in association with gingivitis), fissure sealants, and fluoride applications
- oral health education and promotion
- taking of impressions for, constructing and fitting mouthguards
- referral as necessary to the appropriate practitioner/agency

Department of Health or a New Zealand educational institution. The scope of practice for dental therapists can be found in Box 9-1. In addition to the education and training, the dental therapist can practice independently with consultative supervision, yet very few choose this type of practice setting.

MALAYSIA   There was no dental school in Malaysia until the 1970s, when thirty dentists graduated in 1976. The New Zealand model for educating dental nurses was adopted in Malaysia in 1949. Currently, there are over 2,000 dental nurses. All are female and practice only in primary and secondary school settings. In the school setting, dental nurses are allowed to provide comprehensive dental care to 90% of the children up to age 17. They are not allowed to work in private practice. Most of them will remain employed with the government in this capacity until retirement age, which is 55 years old.

TANZANIA   In 1955, training began for dental assistants to perform many of the functions now done by dental therapists. It wasn't until 1980 that a school for dental therapists opened. Today, dental therapists in Tanzania are limited to performing emergency extractions, due to the low numbers of dentists, and oral health education. The majority of dental therapists are male versus female. Currently, there are only 110 dentists and 150 dental therapists serving a population of over 38 million in Tanzania.

CANADA   Most of the 300 dental therapists in Canada reside and work in the province of Saskatchewan. The Canadian programs are 2 years in length and began in 1972. Upon graduation, practice settings were government-based programs, public health settings, and community clinics where the therapist could provide services to children up to age 19. In 1987, school-based programs were eliminated and dental therapists are now practicing alongside the dentists in private practice settings.

OTHER NATIONS   Fifty other nations that have some model of dental hygiene or oral health care provider other than a dentist, will follow much of the same education and practice models described above. So as the dental community in United States begins to realize that the need in this country is no less than the others, states will have to change dental practice acts accordingly and allow a broader spectrum of delivering oral health care. Legislative changes are never easy and can take many years. Dental hygiene graduates today have a unique opportunity to get involved and become the driving force behind necessary changes.

Dental Therapists in the United States

Although Alaska began using dental therapists before any other state, and Colorado, New Mexico, California, and others have begun education and licensing alternative practice dental hygienists, Minnesota has to be credited for designing curriculum and beginning the two programs that are likely to contribute to the advancement of dental hygienists and the future of oral health care delivery. Minnesota is one state among many that has vast rural areas with little or no access to traditional dental care. As a result, the Minnesota legislators have supported alternate educational programs and practice laws that address opportunities to decrease disparities in their state. In addition to legislative support, professional organizations such as the American Dental Association (ADA), the American Dental Hygienists' Association (ADHA), and the American Dental Educators' Association (ADEA), are supporting the new workforce models that have begun at University of Minnesota and Normandale Community College in association with Metropolitan State University, St. Paul. These models are only the beginning of what might be determined as a paradigm shift in both dental and dental hygiene education and alternative practice.

Minnesota—The Advanced Dental Therapist

Minnesota's version of ADHA's Advanced Dental Hygiene Practitioner (ADHP) model is the *advanced dental therapist (ADT)*. The credit goes to Colleen Brickle, RDH, Ed.D., and interim dean of health sciences at Normandale Community College, who states, "This is one step toward health reform that addresses those who need oral health care the most." Dental hygiene can join in and celebrate Minnesota's victory and realize there are a number of states hoping to follow Minnesota's lead.

In 2008, the ADHA developed educational competencies for the ADHP model in hopes that existing dental hygiene programs would be able to add a new educational path. However, it was state practice acts that became the major barrier to alternative practice models. So, on May 13, 2009, Minnesota Governor Tim Pawlenty signed Senate File 2083, establishing as a law the advanced dental therapist, making Minnesota the first state to pass legislation allowing a **mid-level oral health provider** (dentistry's version of a nurse practitioner).

The ADT program is offered through a collaborative partnership between Normandale Community College and Metropolitan State University. There are two dental hygiene degree completion programs offered with emphasis on collaborative and advanced dental hygiene practice: the baccalaureate degree completion in dental hygiene (BSDH) and the post-baccalaureate certificate in collaborative and advanced dental hygiene practice. For the master's degree as an oral health care practitioner, the curriculum includes higher levels of community-based oral health delivery, collaborative agreements, pharmacology, epidemiology, and medical emergencies. A total of 44 credits are required for graduation, and prospective students have to meet specific prerequisites.

For the baccalaureate degree, the design of this program is based on Minnesota legislation called "Limited Authorization of Dental Hygienists" commonly referred to as "collaborative agreements." This legislation allows the dental hygienist to practice in alternative settings once a formal agreement between a dentist and dental hygienist is established. One goal of this program is to graduate students who are community-minded oral health care providers. Three of the courses included in the degree completion program are required for admission into the master of science: Oral Health Care Practitioner (www.metrostate.edu, 2010). The scope of practice for the ADT is briefly described in Box 9-2.

As shown in Box 9-2, the scope of practice for addressing oral health care disparities has expanded significantly. The official components required for a collaborative agreement in Minnesota includes but it not limited to: identifying the practice settings, emergency plans, listing any limitations on services performed by the ADT, and patient referral criteria. For more information on the ADT and scope of practice visit the website of the Minnesota Office of the Revisor of Statutes (https://www.revisor.mn.gov/statutes/?id=150A).

Dental Therapist

In 2009, the University of Minnesota (U of M) School of Dentistry became the first dental school in the nation to create an educational program for dental therapists. Students enter the University of Minnesota dental therapist program after completing one year of prerequisite college coursework, which includes sciences such as biology, biochemistry, and chemistry along with psychology.

The dental therapist program offered by U of M is unique in that the dental therapy students are taking the same courses as the dental students and the dental hygiene students. The scope of practice will be the same as shown in Box 9-2. The year-round program in dental therapy allows students to complete a bachelor of science degree in 40 months, providing maximum opportunities for those eager to start their dental therapy careers (www.dentistry.umn.edu, 2010).

Alaska—Dental Health Aide Therapists

Because of the prevalence of severe dental disease among Alaska Native children and the chronic shortage of dentists in Alaska, the Alaska Native Tribal Health Consortium (ANTHC), in 2003, with the support of the Indian Health Service, sent six Alaskans to be trained as dental therapists at the University of Otago, Dunedin, New Zealand's national dental school. They returned to Alaska in 2005 to begin caring for patients, primarily children, in rural villages and were sued by the ADA to stop what the association considered to be the illegal practice of dentistry (Nash, 2009). Today, there are 11 dental therapists in practice.

Presently, the Alaska Native Tribal Health Consortium (ANTHC) has established DEN-TEX, in collaboration with the University of Washington School of Medicine Physician

BOX 9-2

Advanced Dental Therapist Scope of Practice

Scope of Practice

An advanced dental therapist certified by the board under this section may perform the following services and procedures pursuant to the written collaborative management agreement:

   (a) an oral evaluation and assessment of dental disease and
   (b) the formulation of an individualized treatment plan authorized by the collaborating dentist;

     The services authorized to be performed by a licensed dental therapist include the oral health services, as specified in paragraphs (c) and (d), and *within the parameters of the collaborative management agreement.*

   (c) A licensed dental therapist may perform the following services under general supervision, unless restricted or
     prohibited in the collaborative management agreement:
     (1) oral health instruction and disease prevention education, including nutritional counseling and dietary analysis;
     (2) preliminary charting of the oral cavity;
     (3) making radiographs;
     (4) mechanical polishing;
     (5) application of topical preventive or prophylactic agents, including fluoride varnishes and pit and fissure sealants;
     (6) pulp vitality testing;
     (7) application of desensitizing medication or resin;
     (8) fabrication of athletic mouthguards;
     (9) placement of temporary restorations;
     (10) fabrication of soft occlusal guards;
     (11) tissue conditioning and soft reline;
     (12) atraumatic restorative therapy;
     (13) dressing changes;
     (14) tooth reimplantation;
     (15) administration of local anesthetic; and
     (16) administration of nitrous oxide.

   (d) A licensed dental therapist may perform the following services under indirect supervision:
     (1) emergency palliative treatment of dental pain;
     (2) the placement and removal of space maintainers;
     (3) cavity preparation;
     (4) restoration of primary and permanent teeth;
     (5) placement of temporary crowns;
     (6) preparation and placement of preformed crowns;
     (7) pulpotomies on primary teeth;
     (8) indirect and direct pulp capping on primary and permanent teeth;
     (9) stabilization of reimplanted teeth;
     (10) extractions of primary teeth;
     (11) suture removal;
     (12) brush biopsies;
     (13) repair of defective prosthetic devices; and
     (14) recementing of permanent crowns.

Source: Minnesota Office of the Revisor of Statutes 150A.106, 150A.105, 2010.

Assistant Training Program, MEDEX Northwest (http://www.washington.edu/medicine/som/depts/medex/). DENTEX is committed to training Alaska Native dental health professionals to practice dental therapy with dentist supervision. The program provides a focused, competency-based, primary care curriculum emphasizing community-level dental disease prevention for underserved Alaska Native populations. The curriculum incorporates innovative public health–related preventive and clinical strategies to address the vast unmet needs of the Alaska Native population (Alaska Native Tribal Health Consortium, 2010).

The first class consisting of three students, graduated from the program on December 12, 2008. This was the nation's first ever group of U.S.-trained dental health aide therapists (DHAT). The second class, which consisted of six students, graduated on December 11, 2009. Class three consists of seven students in their second year of training at the Yuut Elitnaurivat Dental Training Clinic in Bethel, and they are expected to graduate on December 10, 2010. As of March 2010 they've treated over 300 patients.

The need in Alaska was determined to be so great, that developing the DHAT program was nearly the only option to improve oral health in the many rural towns in the state. Now, with the few who have graduated, Alaska has the opportunity to make a difference in the oral health care options for children and families. Seeing a need and a way to meet it as the ANTCH did is the beginning of a new vision for oral healthcare providers and is one more path in the career for dental hygienists.

CURRENT ALTERNATIVE PRACTICE MODELS IN THE UNITED STATES

California

California began the most significant movement toward alternative practice in the mid-1980s. After 10 years of the Health Manpower project, practicing dental hygienists such as Judy Boothby, along with dental hygiene educators, developed the curriculum that would lead to the current registered dental hygienist in alternative practice (RDHAP) programs offered and the University of the Pacific, San Francisco (UOP), and West Los Angeles Community College (WLAC). The 21 dental hygienists who participated in the Health Manpower Project were "grandfathered" into RDHAP licensure, and Boothby has the honor of holding license number one (RDHAP #1). Boothby is respected as the major force behind the success of getting legislators to listen and understand the need for alternative practice in dental hygiene. Alongside Boothby were other major players such as the legislative council of the California Dental Hygienists' Association and their lobbyists Aaron Read and Terry McHale, without whom such success would not have been realized. (Figures 9-1, 9-2, 9-3, and 9-4).

EDUCATION CRITERIA   For practicing dental hygienists interested in taking the next step to becoming a RDHAP, the education and practical experience criteria must be determined. Box 9-3 represents the minimum requirements for application to a program.

The focus of the RDHAP curriculum includes: information management; dental hygiene practice; medically complex patients; oral pathology; pharmacology; developmental disabilities and oral health care; geriatrics; medical and dental emergencies; business administration for dental hygienists; treatment for children with and without special needs; case studies and a community field assignment (www.dental.pacific.edu, 2010).

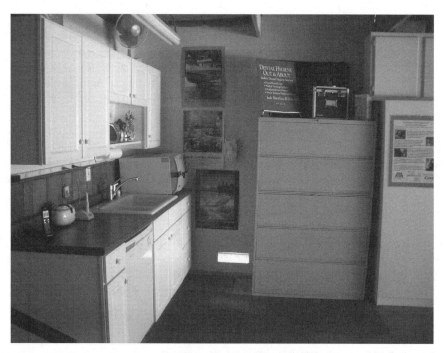

FIGURE 9-1   Boothby's sterilization and instrument storage area situated in the garage.

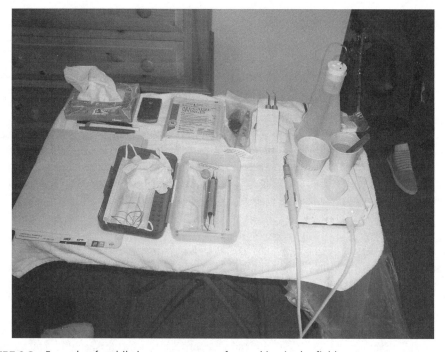

FIGURE 9-2   Example of mobile instrument set-up for working in the field.

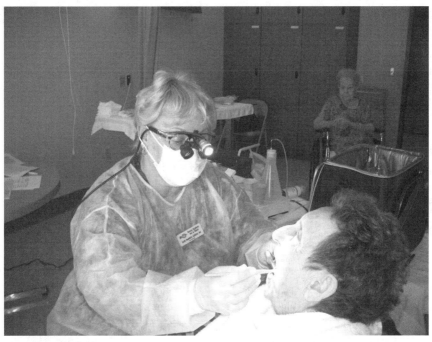

FIGURE 9-3   Judy Boothby providing chair-side care for her patient in the nursing facility.

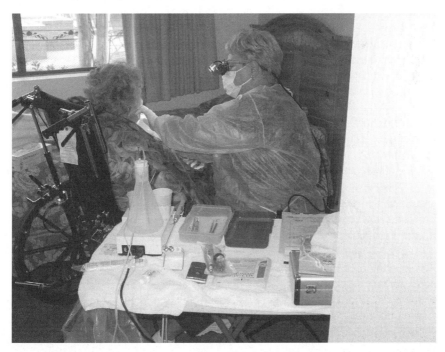

FIGURE 9-4   Taking dental hygiene services to the patient who cannot access care in a traditional dental office.

BOX 9-3

Entrance Requirements for RDHAP Programs in California

1. Hold a current Registered Dental Hygienist license;
2. Have been engaged in clinical practice as a dental hygienist for a minimum of 2,000 hours during the immediately preceding 36 months (which can be in California or another state);
3. Possess a bachelor's degree or its equivalent;
4. Complete 150 hours of an approved educational program; and
5. Pass a written examination prescribed by the dental board.

Upon meeting the criteria identified in Box 9-3, the dental hygienist is eligible for either RDHAP programs: UOP or WLAC. One advantage for the practicing dental hygienist is that the 4-month UOP program is delivered online with a class meeting at the start and end of the program. For those who prefer face-to-face instruction and more interaction with faculty, the WLAC program may fit best.

PRESCRIPTIVE RELATIONSHIPS   After obtaining the alternative practice license (AP), the practitioner has the opportunity to develop prescriptive relationships with dentists in their community that will allow the AP to plan and implement a practice targeting the group they are most interested, such as the geriatric. An RDHAP is allowed to provide services without a prescription 18 months after which, he or she must obtain a written verification that the patient has been examined by a dentist, or physician and surgeon before providing additional dental hygiene services. The dentist or medical doctor then includes a prescription for the continuation of dental hygiene services. The new prescription remains valid for 2 years.

OWNING A PRACTICE   Once professional relationships are established with dentists and or a medical doctor, the RDHAP has to opportunity to build a practice and deliver oral health care to target populations he or she is most interested. Many choose to target the elderly, homebound persons, and the mentally or physically challenged. Yet, there are still many areas of California where the RDHAP can make a difference, which may include migrant workers or rural children and families. As an RDHAP, creating the kind of practice you may envision has resulted from numerous dedicated professionals who worked to ensure the future of dental hygienists and improve access to quality oral health care.

Prior to the establishment of an independent practice, an RDHAP must provide the dental board documentation of an existing relationship with at least one dentist for referral, consultation, and emergency services. The dentist's license must be current, active, and not under discipline by the board. Any changes in the relationship must be reported to the board in writing, within 30 days following such change.

As an RDHAP, the scope of practice now includes:

• Residences of the homebound
• Schools

- Residential facilities and other institutions
- Dental health professional shortage areas, as certified by the Office of Statewide Health Planning and Development in accordance with existing office guidelines

With a few more months of education, the RDHAP is one more way the dental hygienist can make a difference in the oral health of those who cannot access the traditional dental practice setting. After gaining practical experience as a dental hygienist, alternative practice may be a direction of interest in the future.

Colorado—Unsupervised Practice

In 1987, Colorado dental hygiene gained notoriety allowing unsupervised dental hygiene practice, which lead to one version of independent practice. The 2009 Dental Practice Law in Colorado defines unsupervised practice as "unless licensed to practice dentistry, a person shall be deemed to be practicing unsupervised dental hygiene who, within the scope of the person's education, training, and experience . . ." would include specific duties such as those common to dental hygiene practice, however the unsupervised practitioner can apply sealants, topical anesthetic, fluoride varnish, and antimicrobial solutions. The law also states the dental hygienist can perform a dental hygiene diagnosis, determine a dental hygiene treatment plan, and is required to refer patients for a dental examination twice a year. Radiographs and administration of local anesthetic and nitrous oxide sedation still requires direct supervision; therefore, those practicing unsupervised will need to maintain positive relationships with the dental community to work collaboratively in the best interest of the patient.

CONTINUED OPPOSITION   In 1998, a pilot study of six independent practicing dental hygienists was conducted by Astroth and Cross-Poline to determine productivity and service mix as compared to those practicing in traditional office settings. They concluded the care provided was consistent with the care provided with those who participated in the Health Manpower Pilot Project #139, in California. There were no undue risks to the safety and health of the public being served by these practitioners (Winter, 1998).

Despite the fact that dental hygienists gain appropriate education, training, licensure, and adhere to a code of ethics and moral values, the dental community does not see the benefit of unsupervised or independent practice for dental hygienists. In 2005, an article published in the *Journal of the American Dental Association* (JADA), pointed out that only 20 of the 2,700 dental hygienists were practicing independently (Berry, 2005). The argument for dentistry is that the low number of dental hygienists choosing to practice independently is not improving the access to care problem. However, as the ADHA pointed out in a written response, Colorado is not the only state providing a model of unsupervised practice. When more states change laws regarding dental hygiene practice then the public gains better access to preventive and therapeutic services provided by dental hygienists (ADHA, 2005).

Maine—Unsupervised Practice

Maine began changing access to care laws by passing expanded functions for both dental assistants and dental hygienists. In 2007, Maine legislators enacted HP0309, LD 421, which established criteria for education and experience to become an unsupervised independent practitioner. Since then, Maine has adopted legislation that will allow these practitioners to receive direct reimbursement for services provided. Additionally, owning radiographic equipment is now included allowing the dental hygienist to produce sufficient records to establish the dental hygiene diagnosis and treatment plan. The changes in Maine's law is so new that some of the new rules and regulations will not be enacted until October 2010, therefore are not found in the current edition of the Dental Practice Act. However, this opportunity truly may be setting the stage for the other 18 states to seek more legislative changes and continue the forward movement for dental hygiene.

New Mexico—Collaborative Practice

The New Mexico statute defines collaborative dental hygiene practitioner as a hygienist who is certified by the New Mexico Board of Dental Health Care and Dental Hygienists' Committee to provide dental hygiene services, except for local anesthesia, without general supervision, in a cooperative working relationship with a dentist. The scope of services that a dental hygienist can provide remains the same (New Mexico Dental Hygienists' Association, 2010). The change in dental hygiene practice was recommended by the New Mexico Health Policy Commission as a result of a study by a task force comprised of various health care professionals. The task force recognized that dental hygienists were an underutilized provider, limited by restrictions in the state statute. By removing supervision requirements, collaborative hygienists are able to work in various health care settings, providing dental hygiene services to many who would not otherwise have access to care (New Mexico Dental Hygienists' Association, 2010).

IS IT WORKING?   Collaborative practice has been in place for 5 years. It is certainly an entry point for many New Mexico citizens into the dental care system. The dental community may indicate that the impact of collaborative practice has not been significant but consumers who now receive basic preventive services would disagree. Because collaborative hygienists partner with a consulting dentist who provides further diagnostic and restorative care for the patients, collaborative practice can be a beneficial situation for everyone. Collaborative practice will continue to evolve and reach even more people needing basic preventive oral health care services (New Mexico Dental Hygienists' Association, 2010).

Case Study Follow-up #2

Using the information for the scope of dental hygiene practice in your state, are they different from those described for the dental therapist, RDHAP, collaborative practice, and unsupervised practice in Maine?

Summary

The education and career choices for dental hygienists has entered a new phase, and rightfully so. In 1898, Dr. M.L. Rhein employed a woman he called a dental nurse to perform what become known as the oral prophylaxis in his office. In 1903, Dr. Rhein proposed formal education for dental nurses, and in 1903 Dr. Alfred C. Fones trained Irene Newman, who became the first licensed dental hygienist in 1917 (Darby & Walsh, 1998). During the development of dental hygiene education and practice, supervision by the dentist was inherent. However, it has now been 112 years since Dr. Rhein began thinking outside of the box, and supervision remains the largest barrier for both consumers and dental hygiene professionals.

Dental hygienists are not dentists, yet their education can span the same number of years or more as dentistry. Dental hygienists are increasingly seeking masters and doctoral degrees in an array of areas: dental hygiene, public health, administration, politics, education, and research. The practice of dental hygiene is no longer limited to the dental office and continues to expand through forward-thinking practitioners and legislators. The consumer needs to be the focus of attention when it comes to improved oral health, not the supervision issue. By altering this mindset, the public has the opportunity to gain access to care in a variety of ways, and improve their overall health.

Alternative practice choices like those in California, Maine, Minnesota, Alaska, and New Mexico are making the difference for all dental hygiene professionals. No longer is the dental hygiene graduate relegated to a private practice setting for their entire career. Along with the six roles of the dental hygienist, alternative practice can be added as another pathway for all those who choose clinical practice. The future of dental hygiene will continue to evolve. It is an evolutionary process of necessity and will require dental hygienists to continue with higher education in order to effectively make changes in legislation and scope of practice.

Critical Thinking

1. Describe the education differences between the dental therapist and the dental hygienist.
2. What are the qualifications for application to a RDHAP program?
3. Why does it appear that the dental community does not support alternative practice models for dental hygienists?
4. When thinking about alternative practice, outline what it will take to start your own practice (equipment, supplies, funding, etc). Who might be your target population? What type of practice might you prefer (mobile, collaborative, dental therapist)? Use your outline with the information for developing a business plan located on MyHealthProfessionsKit and begin a business plan for an alternative practice.
5. If your state does not allow some version of limited supervision or unsupervised practice for dental hygienists, what are some of the ways to begin changing the laws?

CHAPTER 10

Seeking the Dental Hygiene Position

OBJECTIVES

After reading the material in this chapter, you will be able to

- Discuss aspects of *job searching*.
- Identify different *employment opportunities* for dental hygienists.
- Discuss the *process of interviews* between employers and employees.
- Identify the advantages and disadvantages of *working interviews*.
- Identify contents and needs for office *policy manuals*.
- Discuss *benefits* as they relate to the dental hygienist.
- Apply *negotiating skills* related to employee benefits.

KEY TERMS

Benefits	Evaluations	Policy manuals
Cost of living	Merit	Résumé

INTRODUCTION

Upon graduation, dental hygienists begin to look at what it will to take to find the right position. Many students relocate from their home community to attend dental hygiene school. Oftentimes, they decide to stay in the new location rather than return home to begin a career. Searching for a job after graduation requires some research and planning.

There can be several options for employment as graduates begin to interview for positions. A working interview has become very common because it allows both the graduate and the office staff to become familiar with each other. Depending on where you want to begin your career, there will be employment resources available to assist in the search. Interviews for new graduates can be daunting if they are unprepared. Not only will the dentist interview you, you will want to be prepared to interview your potential employer. Developing a set of questions for the dentist will be just as important as any question he or she may ask of you. Your résumé should already be updated and provided to the dentist when you first meet. It will also provide a good starting point for an interview exchange.

This chapter will discuss many aspects of seeking a new dental hygiene position, including how to prepare for interviews and the expectations that employers, coworkers, and patients establish for new faces in the practice. As new graduates begin their career, they need to understand how compensation works for dental hygienists and where potential negotiating points could land a great benefit package. The chapter also points out essential workplace documents such as policy manuals and employment contracts.

Case Study

The practice you have been employed in for 8 years has been sold to a new dentist following the retirement of your employer. The new dentist has met with the employees as a group and announced that she has reviewed the employee benefits package and salary scale and that, on the recommendation of the accountant and the consultant, the benefit package must be modified. She has implied that some benefits may be reduced by 40% or some areas cut in order to improve the practice profits.

The employees called a meeting to discuss the possible reduction of the benefits package and to develop a way to keep the package.

As you read this chapter, consider the following: How would you outline a benefit package for the employees that will satisfy everyone? On the basis of your package, identify items that are negotiable and prepare to negotiate with the dentist at the next meeting.

BEGINNING THE SEARCH

New graduates should investigate open positions within their community, the surrounding communities, and practices that have difficulty getting dental hygienists to consider their offer. Whether the educational program you attended is located in an urban or a rural area, you need to look at several factors that may help to determine where to begin practice.

Surveys done by the American Dental Association (ADA) indicate that there is a shortage of dental hygienists in certain parts of the country. This may be partially true since there are areas where dental hygienists do not reside. However, employment surveys conducted by the American Dental Hygienists' Association (ADHA) indicate that a maldistribution of dental hygienists may be more accurate. This means that the dental hygienists may be plentiful in urban communities, while rural areas experience a lack of clinicians to provide dental hygiene services. This may be a result of dental hygienists being unwilling to relocate or commute to surrounding areas. Another possible reason for lack of open positions may stem from dental hygienists choosing to stay in permanent positions within their communities. Dental hygiene can be a very flexible career. Many hygienists will have the opportunity to work as much or as little as they like. Additionally, many practitioners are satisfied with their positions and their employers; thus, shifting in dental hygiene positions will not happen frequently. Should this occur in the area where you reside, relocation to a community where dental hygiene positions are more abundant may be the next-best alternative.

Keep Options Open

Many dental hygienists are unable to relocate, however, because of family ties and commitments, but commuting is an option to consider. A 30-minute drive one way to work can be a long distance for some, while for others commuting means at least 45 to 60 minutes or more. Regardless of the distance, the time it takes to commute to work is another factor to consider when searching for a position. Commuting to outlying communities is another opportunity to gain employment more quickly if relocation is not an option. Overnight stays may decrease the expense of the commute, wear and tear on the vehicle, and fuel costs, and the dental hygienist may be able to work two or three days in the same office. This can be advantageous because the opportunity to acquire an immediate position may be easier, and new graduates are providing preventive oral health care to an area that may have difficulty getting dental hygienists to commute or relocate. These factors may be negotiating points with the employer and are discussed later in this chapter.

WORKING AS A TEMPORARY

Temporary employment is another good option for an immediate position if the dental hygienist resides in an area where job openings occur less frequently. Furthermore, this can be an excellent source of steady, yet flexible employment. Many practices are opting to schedule advance appointments for dental hygiene patients. This means that the dental hygienist can be scheduled 3 to 6 months in advance. Unless vacations are preblocked in the schedule, the dental hygienist may find it difficult to take time off from work. In addition, when time off is taken in the hygiene department, the practice may see a decrease in production and collections since fewer patients are scheduled.

One way to alleviate downtime for the practice is to hire a *temporary* during regular staff vacations or extended periods of absence, such as maternity leaves. By doing this, the practice makes a positive business decision because it will not have to reschedule patients. Temporary employees have the opportunity to work in many environments for short periods.

DENTAL EMPLOYMENT AGENCIES   Many communities have agencies that specialize in dental personnel, offering the new graduate the opportunity to market himself or herself as a temporary employee. Working with a temporary agency is another way to gain employment, and for many, working as a temp is a viable source of regular employment and income. The value of marketing and public relations skills is certainly applicable to this type of situation. Compensation may be handled differently under temporary positions, so consult a tax accountant on what is expected for temporary employment.

ADVANTAGES AND DISADVANTAGES   There are many advantages to beginning a new career in a temporary position. The new practitioner is able to test numerous dental practices. When unsure as to what type of office environment you seek, temporary positions will allow you to work with many offices, their staff members, and their patients. This way, if the environment is not compatible with the way you had planned on practicing your discipline, it becomes easy to move on to the next position.

The disadvantage is that there may be times when the clinician is unsure as to when the next position will present itself. However, this may be a small inconvenience when evaluating the advantages.

EMPLOYMENT RESOURCES

New graduates may be unfamiliar with where or how to seek employment. The following resources are likely available in your area and will assist you in getting started in a career search:

- *Dental practices* Many dental practices will submit flyers to dental hygiene programs and request placement on the career bulletin board. This is one resource to investigate before leaving school.
- *ADHA* As mentioned, seeking career information through the ADHA is the first step to finding the position that suits each dental hygienist.
- *The Internet* The Internet is fast becoming a valuable resource for numerous needs in the career industry (key words: "job search").
- *Other resources* Other resources include state and local dental hygiene organizations, local dental organizations, practicing professionals, dental assistants, the classified ads, professional journal advertisements, and employment agencies, your school website, and job connection websites.

PREPARING FOR INTERVIEWS

After taking clinical board examinations and prior to receiving a license to practice, dental hygiene graduates may be interviewing with potential employers in areas they think they may want to practice. During interviews with possible employers, many new graduates are so overwhelmed at beginning their new career that they often miss information being presented and the opportunity to ask important questions that may help them understand what a new employer expects. When entering a practice for a scheduled interview, the applicant immediately notices the environment, the office decor, the atmosphere, and how modern the equipment may be. Often, a new dental hygienist visualizes himself or herself in the new working environment and wants to be sure that he or she will be comfortable in that particular environment. Providing dental hygiene services, education, and motivation to patients in each practice is the basis of the education and training. However, during that interview process, numerous subjects may not be discussed because of time constraints (the dentist may be interviewing during working hours and between patients) or because neither party is fully prepared to discuss important information related to the open position. Most important, employers have expectations that new dental hygienists may not be aware of. Many of these expectations underlie the association of employees with the practice and often go unrealized. When initiating a career search, endless hours will be spent if the search is to be successful. Each interview becomes critical in moving forward to the goal of that first position. For those who interview frequently, job offers should be expected. If the résumés and letters of interest are not getting you an interview, then reevaluation of the search strategy becomes necessary. Preparation is essential to eliminating stress.

Interviewing Skills

Interviewing skills are key factors in selecting the person who will fit into a practice. The main purpose of interviewing is for the dental hygienist and the potential employer to learn about each other. Formats range from telephone interviews to panel interviews to personal settings. No matter the form, the process remains similar.

BOX 10-1

Effective Interviewing Techniques

Be Proactive

Essentially, this means to take initiative and responsibility for yourself. Generally, most people are reactive to their surroundings and the things that happen to them. With increased knowledge in business and management, being proactive allows you to stand out and be seen as a leader. Being proactive in an interview situation, the new employee would initiate pertinent questions applicable to duties that may be performed if employed with the office. For example, dentists generally ask how a dental hygienist determines the need for root planing procedures. When taking a proactive approach to interview questions, the employee might be the one to ask how the office determines root planing procedures and what the policy is for referrals to a specialist.

Begin with the End in Mind

Where do you want to be next year at this time? What type of practice do you want to be associated with? Some things to consider when interviewing include the following:

- Informal/formal environment
- Casual personalities
- Open communication
- Oral health care philosophy

Knowing what type of environment you want to be working in at a future date will help you decide in what type of practice you want to work.

The Win-Win Outcome

Many new graduates may not be hired after an interview and feel as though they lost to someone who may have had better qualifications. When interviewees are not hired, there is always something gained from the interview, because it is a learning experience. Covey (1990) explains that the win-win situation is a frame of heart and mind seeking the benefit of all interactions (p. 207). So, no matter the outcome, there is a learned experience that becomes incorporated into each person's background that may be of benefit at a later point.

It is important to be prepared with your own expectations and questions when interviewing with potential employers. What is the best approach to interviews when seeking the first or the tenth career position? Taking the interview process in steps will help the applicant anticipate questions that may be asked by employers and prepare questions to ask of prospective employers. Using some principles of Stephen R. Covey's habits from *The 7 Habits of Highly Effective People*, we can see how certain aspects may be applied to dental hygiene interview techniques. See Box 10-1 for a list of effective interviewing techniques.

Interviewing can be an arduous task for the practice and a nerve-racking experience for a new dental hygiene graduate. By taking the time to incorporate appropriate information and develop new tools that can be of use, all experiences have a positive outcome.

The Employer's Interview

Selecting the right person for employment is a skill that may take years to develop. Employers become frustrated when the turnover rate in their practice is high and they go through employees every 6 months. Changes in any practice can be expensive, annoying, and frustrating to each staff member. For new dental hygiene graduates, having an understanding of what the employer must consider will be of benefit when preparing for interviews.

EMPLOYER RESPONSIBILITIES   Some considerations by the employer may include the following:

- Determining the level of competency needed for the open position
- Preparing a job description to orient the new employee
- Explaining the job requirements during the interview
- Accurately observing the person being interviewed
- Evaluating the responses from the prospective employee

LEGAL CONSIDERATIONS   In addition, the employer and potential employee must be aware of the legal aspects of the interview process. Every state has laws against discrimination. These laws must also be adhered to during interviews. Questions in an interview process cannot include the following:

- Those related to race or color
- Those related to gender or religion
- Those related to marital status, age, or the number of children one may have
- Those related to military status
- Those related to national origin or residency

(In 1986, the Immigration Reform and Control Act specified requirements for new employees to complete an I-9 form. This form was designed to prevent the employment of illegal aliens.)

Social security numbers are also matters of personal information. Many organizations have begun to eliminate the use of social security numbers as a form of identification, opting for use of randomly selected numbers. Now that some groundwork has been explained and defined, what types of questions could an employer ask, and what might the employer be looking for in a new employee? How might the actual interview take place? Most employers will do their best to keep the interview relaxed and comfortable. This helps bring out true personalities and may encourage more self-disclosure from both parties.

Common Interview Questions

Questions regarding personal and professional behavior are typically used to initiate the session:

- How would you describe yourself in a working environment?
- Why do you feel you would like to work with this practice?
- Why did you leave your last position?
- Can you handle constructive criticism?
- How would you handle questions about fees from your patients?
- How would you handle an irate patient?
- What salary range are you expecting?
- What specialized qualifications or education do you possess?

Of course, each employer and each interview will be unique. Some interviews will include the business or office manager, and some are handled exclusively by either. This is similar to a screening technique. If the office manager conducts interviews, the employer may reinterview only when the potential candidates have been selected.

During each interview, be sure to listen carefully to the questions being asked. Answers should focus on your qualifications, special skills, and education. You may focus on aspects dental hygiene courses that you feel contributed to your strong points or that held a particular interest for you. Make sure to emphasize the potential benefits you feel you can bring to the practice. Interjecting personal information is fine but be sure not to dwell too long on the topic.

THE APPLICANT'S ATTITUDE   Employers expect a positive attitude in any prospective employee. Promptness is observed the first time you enter the practice. Do not arrive late for any interview.

Your Interview

While in dental hygiene school, many students envision what they would like as they begin their careers. What will the appointments be like? Will new graduates be given a full hour for each appointment, or does the practice expect the entering dental hygienist to manage within the same time as the person who has been with the practice for several years? Does everyone expect to begin his or her new career in the ideal working environment? A good option for answers to these questions is to shadow the dental hygienist in the office for few hours. Shadowing allows you to observe the office in action.

OUTLINING EXPECTATIONS   As interviews begin, new licensees will want to develop an outline of their own expectations or perhaps of the environment in which they prefer to work. Salary is likely the most common topic on the minds of both the employer and the applicant. Yet if questions arise on what you expect as a starting wage, you will want to have a figure ready to present to the dentist or potential employer. Research this figure through various avenues. Contact the state local dental hygiene association for the most recent information on salary ranges in your area. There will be many topics such as this that you will want to research. Be prepared with pertinent questions for the employer so that accepting a position is based on complete information about the practice and the duties expected of you.

INTERVIEW QUESTIONS TO AVOID   How about questions to ask the employer? In order to present yourself professionally, there are also questions you should avoid. For example, do not:

- Ask what they can offer you
- Ask what the top pay rate is in the office
- Ask if your schedule can be altered for your child's after-school activities
- State that you have no questions at all

Skill and technique are important when beginning to interview. Many interviews contribute to improving skills.

Another aspect to avoid is appearing desperate for a position. When new practitioners present themselves in this manner, they are likely to engage certain pitfalls of employment, including a lower-than-average wage, fewer benefits if applicable, fewer workdays, or perhaps longer working hours. These things can happen to anyone when unprepared. Examples of questions to ask the interviewer include those found in Box 10-2.

BOX 10-2

Sample Interview Questions

Clinical Concerns

- What kinds of instruments are used in the office?
- Is the employer willing to order instruments?
- Are instruments shared among the dental hygienists in the office?
- Who makes the dental hygiene diagnosis and treatment plan?
- What is the protocol for referrals to specialists?
- What sterilization methods are employed?
- To what extent are Occupational Safety and Health Administration (OSHA) standards practiced?

Scheduling

- Who schedules dental hygiene appointments?
- What recall system is practiced?
- What is expected when patients fail appointments?
- How long are hygiene appointments? (forty-five or sixty minutes)

General Practice Information

- What constitutes full time and part time?
- What is the negotiable salary range?
- Does the office pay for continuing education courses?
- How is the computer system applied to hygiene services?
- What benefits are available to the dental hygienist?
- Does the staff work when the dentist is out of the office?
- How interactive are staff meetings, and how often are they held?
- What is the channel of communication or command?

These are only some of the questions new graduates can incorporate into an interview. Keep in mind that presenting yourself as an experienced professional will be advantageous to potential employers. Thus, planning for questions is essential to the overall presentation. Communicating with dental hygienists who work or have worked in the office is recommended, as they can offer another perspective on the operations and working personalities of the practice. In the employment interview, questions from new graduates are valid and will assist in making the decision to become employed in that particular office.

The Working Interview

Employers will often want to try the dental hygienist before actually hiring him or her on a permanent basis. Working interviews may consist of one full or half day or even a few weeks of providing clinical services to the patients. The dental hygienist is compensated for these services and will want to fully understand when the pay period occurs and how much the pay will be for the period agreed on.

ADVANTAGES FOR BOTH PARTIES Advantages of a working interview for the employer include being able to indirectly observe clinical skills, interpersonal skills with patients, and relationship skills with coworkers. The advantages for the dental hygienist include being able to observe how the staff interact with them and others, how staff interact with patients, and how everyone interacts with the employer. Another advantage for the dental hygienist is that he or she is able to work with the equipment and instruments that are currently in the practice. This will provide information on what may need replacement or must be purchased should he or she decide to take this position. He or she can also determine whether the time allotment for each patient is sufficient and whether there is pressure to stay on time. How receptive is the staff to questions when the new employee is uncertain of office procedures or locating materials?

Working interviews may be more of an advantage than one may think. Most new employees are excited about being hired for a permanent position, only to realize a few weeks later that working philosophies do not mesh or that other negative issues exist. New practitioners have nothing to lose, as compensation is given for their time. When unsure as to whether to accept a position, suggest a working interview to the employer.

Interviews and Personality Tests

Although rare, there are employers who have applicants take a personality test. Not all personality tests are written. Some are oral; thus, you may be unaware this test is being given. Personality tests are designed to assist in identifying certain behaviors, habits, or patterns held by a person. Oral interviews can consist of specific questions that have been designed to promote certain responses from the applicant. Thus, the employer is able to determine your capacity to fit into his or her practice on the basis of your responses. If the employer has used the same technique on every employee hired, the personality of the practice becomes homogeneous in nature, which may make a smooth working environment. As with other aspects associated with job searching, personality tests will also have advantages and disadvantages. When thoroughly prepared for interviews, the professional personality will be expressed naturally.

Attire

Now that some time has been spent getting all the professional information ready to present to potential employers, what clothing is most appropriate for interviews? There are no absolutes for proper dress. However, keep in mind the environment in which the interview will take place. If you are meeting the employer during office hours, you may choose to wear something more professional. This does not mean that clinic attire is required.

CONSIDER INTERVIEWS AS A BUSINESS MEETING Most often, a businesslike approach is best. A business suit makes a professional statement. More and more, dentists may be dropping the white shirt and tie for casual polo shirts or scrubs. However, as a potential new employee, a professional approach makes a better impression. Avoid wearing an outfit if you question its appropriateness: sundresses, sandals, and so on. Stick to slacks, blouses, sweaters, skirts, business dresses, or jackets. Men may opt for shirts and ties.

PERSONAL APPEARANCE Grooming is another factor where image will be represented. If you feel good, you will look good. Pay attention to hairstyles and makeup (for women). Current trends are changing among health care professionals, and many students enter education programs with body art (tattoos), body piercing, and even facial piercing. In addition, seasoned professionals join the trends later in life by adding a tattoo or piercing that may give them their own personal style.

TATTOOS   Body art or tattoos are still controversial simply because of the sterilization processes (or lack thereof) among tattoo artists. There are many tattoo artists who have practiced their craft to the highest degree for decades and are strong advocates for legislation that will establish standard practices for equipment and sterilization among all tattoo artists. In any health care profession, students learn how imperative it is to follow standard precautions and protocol for bloodborne pathogens. Thus, no matter the independent decision to have a new or additional tattoo, there are questions that need to be asked of the artist placing the tattoo. Safety must come first if the licensed clinician chooses to follow cultural trends. If you already have a tattoo that can be seen when dressed for an interview, you may consider covering it. Discussing the dentists' preference or allowance of tattoos may be another interview point to add to your list.

BODY PIERCING   Similar trends are found when it comes to body piercing. Many programs have entering students who have ear cartilage piercing or pierced tragi, noses, tongues, eyebrows, or lips. As many dental hygiene students may be younger, health care careers are finding that these new personal choices may impact the perspective of the consumers. How? Unfortunately, stereotyping still occurs in many nations and cultures. Similar to tattoos, it may be wise to remove body jewelry that is exposed when appropriately attired for an interview. This, too, may be another point of discussion for interviews with potential employers.

CONSUMER PERCEPTION   Dental hygiene education programs work at bringing out the professional in all those who enter the field as licensed health care providers. It is possible that consumers who are receiving treatment by a practitioner with several facial or ear piercings may not be perceived to be as highly qualified as someone who has none. These perceptions may be seen as unfair in the eyes of students and licensed professionals, yet perception can be reality for many consumers. Thus, it is highly possible that most dental hygiene programs do not allow facial piercings, cartilage piercings, or body art to be worn or seen while in the clinic setting or perhaps the program setting.

REPRESENTING THE PRACTICE   What might potential employers perceive of the newly licensed professional who interviews with a pierced nose or eyebrow or the tattoo that may be placed in an area that is seen no matter what clothing is worn? Many dentists may be conservative in their views for their employees. After all, employees interact with their patients every day and are representatives of the practice. Employees are seen as representatives if the dentists' practice. Yet, trends are changing, and many licensed professionals are included in the evolving public perception of body art and body or facial piercings, keep all of these factors in mind as they may have an influence on potential employment.

Everyone has the right to personal choices. However, as a health care provider, be sure to carefully evaluate these choices using newfound or enhanced knowledge of infection control. Additionally, keep in mind that the perception of others may not match the intent of your personal choice; thus, it may be a delicate balancing situation between culture trends and being a licensed health care provider. As graduates seek employment, it may be best to keep it professional or conservative, as in your dental hygiene education. Overall appearance is what the employer and staff observe first. Make a good first impression while feeling confident and comfortable. Neat and clean may be the best approach.

LEADERSHIP VERSUS MANAGEMENT: QUALITIES AND OPPORTUNITIES

Dental hygienists have the opportunity to take on more than just the clinician role in a new office. The office may provide the opportunity to be a leader in projects that occur throughout the year. To help fill their future employee needs, many potential employers look for leadership qualities when they interview new graduates.

So what qualities might a leader possess? And how do they differ from management qualities?

Chapter 7 introduced the three categories of management styles, which are authoritative, free rein, and participatory. Managers are typically held accountable for the total project and expect others to complete their assignments, but do not do all the work. They are responsible for overseeing a project (perhaps the overall goal), may set priorities for achieving steps toward the goal, and often work primarily as a mediator for the project.

As described in Chapter 8, leaders influence, motivate, or direct those around them when working toward a common goal by capturing their interest in the "vision" of the project. Managers accomplish the same goals, but have others do the work.

Leaders have the ability to look at a project that may be done frequently and visualize a new or different way to accomplish the goals. They work to include all parties who may be involved in the project and focus on the overall vision rather than the specific tasks assigned to those working on the project.

Effective leaders are likely to possess some or all of the following characteristics:

- Good time management skills
- Credibility, honesty, and accountability for mistakes
- Good organizational skills, preparedness, and anticipatory skills
- Good communication and listening skills
- Encouraging self-reliance, acknowledging the success of others, and challenging others
- Matching tasks with talents of people (they are innovative)
- Willingness to make decisions, take risks, and recognize failures as experience

A potential employer may ask questions about your leadership qualities at some time during your interview. To be prepared for these questions, use the previous list and the leadership traits identified in Table 8-1 to identify which leadership qualities apply to you as a student, as a graduate, or perhaps in a former employment position. Highlight these leadership qualities in your résumé and be ready to mention these qualities during your interview. By doing so, your qualifications can set you apart from the other job applicants.

Case Study Follow-up #1

List some of the leadership traits you might use as you plan to negotiate the benefits package with the employer.

RÉSUMÉS

Now that you have prepared yourself for the interviews, the next important step is to be sure that your **résumé** is in order. Writing a résumé can be a difficult task, but for many it is the opportunity to identify and promote their talents and skills. Presenting a résumé is presenting a brief statement of employment experience and education. Dental hygiene graduates are able to apply the idea of image in promoting the highest aspects of their qualifications. Many résumé formats are easily found and standard in computer software. Some programs include résumés in word-processing or publishing programs. They are preformatted, so all that is required is filling in the blanks.

PROFESSIONAL FORMAT   A variety of formats, including traditional, professional, and contemporary, allow each person to express individuality. Once created, the résumé can be printed on a high-quality bond paper. Additional resources for résumés are résumé services and local printing or copying businesses as well as the Internet (key word: *"résumé"*). Some firms may have computers available for customers to format their own document. Should a résumé extend longer than one page, there is the possibility that only the first page gets read or the employer skims for pertinent information. Be concise with qualifications but be sure to highlight special aspects that may stand above others applying for the same position.

Résumés should be typed, using a computer, or produced by a professional printer. The font chosen for résumés need to be easily read. Avoid being too elaborate because this can distract from the information presented. Always proofread and reread the final product. Avoid grammatical and spelling errors. Computer programs are extremely useful, but they are not perfect. It is often helpful to have another person proofread the résumé and point out errors or make suggestions when information lacks clarity. How can your résumé stand out among the others?

Perfecting Your Résumé

Focus on the content   If an employer does not have time to read résumés, there is a chance they may quickly glance through the form and decide on whom to interview within a matter of seconds. Past experience can play a major part in such a decision. Highlight your best abilities and accomplishments.

Visual appearance   If the résumé is to get more than a few seconds of attention, it should catch the eye. Color, bullets, borders, spacing, italicizing, and style will add to the presentation of the résumé. Make sure the printer cartridge is new and that the printed résumé is clean.

Be accurate, concise, and clear   List items and accomplishments first so that the reader's attention stays focused. No one wants to search for information that is buried in the "fluff." Interest will be lost quickly, and your résumé may find the shredder. (Box 10-3)

Use an appropriate font and high-quality paper   White, cream, and light blues or grays have shown to be most appealing to readers—nothing fancy, just quality. As mentioned, the font size should be easily read. Font size 12 is widely accepted, but 14 may be too large because it may appear that you are trying to lengthen the document. Font size 10 may be used for sections, but many times it is too small for easy reading.

Proofread and edit   This may be the most difficult task to accomplish. Mistakes are often overlooked because the information is so familiar to the writer. Have someone else proofread for errors and comprehension. Do not send a résumé with typos, spelling errors, or "whiteout" corrections. The goal is perfection and professionalism.

BOX 10-3

Common Résumé Sections

- **Objective statement** This is a brief statement that targets reasons for seeking employment in a particular practice or setting. Usually, it is goal oriented. State the goals you seek on a professional and personal level by being associated with the dentist or practice.
- **Experience** Depending on the amount and scope of experience, include previous jobs that augment the skills required for the new position. Begin with the most recent. Include each employer's name and address and a short description of duties performed in the position.
- **Education** Most important, list all college education, degrees, honors, and awards received. Some may choose to include information on grade-point average; however, it is not necessary. For those who attend special workshops or continuing education seminars that are relevant to the career, it is a good idea to include this information.
- **Professional memberships** If previously licensed or a member of a professional organization, include this in the résumé. This indicates activity and interest in the profession and issues that may affect your career or community.
- **Credentials/licensure** Include all information about your licensure and credentials. If you possess a dental assisting license, list it. Provide the year in which it was received and the license number itself. If you hold other certificates, such as one in cardiopulmonary resuscitation (CPR), be sure to include them. Furthermore, extract any expanded functions affiliated with a dental hygiene license, such as nitrous oxide sedation and local anesthesia. Many states may not include this with the dental hygiene licensure, but if your state does, be sure to highlight those skills.
- **Personal data** It is often advantageous to include information on hobbies, community activities, and family interests. This may give some insight about how you may prioritize aspects of your lifestyle.
- **References** References are generally provided on request. These will include coworkers or personal friends who can attest to your character and to the benefits of having you as an employee. Be sure to select those you prefer to have the potential employer contact, as many employers take the time to call those you have listed.

Résumé styles will differ; however, they will hold the same essential information. The sample résumé in Figure 10-1 represents some of the information that can be incorporated to provide the appropriate information for the position you are seeking to fill. Depending on your past experience and the extent of your education, the résumé will vary in length. Be sure to include all pertinent information, including professional memberships and volunteer programs.

The Cover Letter

A *cover letter* (see Figure 10-2) should accompany your résumé. There are several types of cover letters that can be employed. If the practice has asked for a résumé, the cover letter will want to address the request. If sending résumés as a "cold contact," the focus is on identifying the qualifications needed for the dental hygiene position. Additionally, if someone has referred you to a

Suzanne Anderson, RDH

55 Hilltop Avenue, Riverview   555-0101/sanderson@internet.net

Objective	To actively participate in a progressive oral health environment that promotes quality oral health and provides open communication for new ideas.
Experience	1999–present Kristoffer Leonard, DDS—Periodontics **Clinical Dental Hygienist** Skilled in patient education, digital radiography, scaling and root planing, curettage, and adjunct therapies.
	1998–1999 Rikky Jones, DDS, General Dentistry Southridge, SC **Chairside Assistant** • Four-handed dentistry • OSHA monitor • Clinical inventory
	1997–1999 Samuel Ferguson, DDS, and Charlene O'Connor, DDS Southridge, SC **Insurance Coordinator** • Daily insurance processing/claims
	1995–1997 R. Clark DDS Ridgeport, SC
	1998–2000 Southridge Community College, SC
Education	• A.S. Dental Hygiene—Honors • 1992 BS Biology, Southridge State College, SC LICENSURE: 2006 DH State License #55551. Skilled in clinical aspects of debridement, root planing, local anesthesia, nitrous oxide sedation, sealant placement, periodontal assessment, treatment planning, and patient education. • Master of Science, Health Administration—pending date of graduation May 2004
Professional memberships	Member—American Dental Hygienists' Association South Carolina Dental Hygienists Association Riverview Rotary Club SCC Alumni Association
Community work	• Volunteer for county school screenings • Oral health fairs: elementary schools • Tobacco cessation presentations at local high schools
Interests	Outdoor activities, horseback riding, water sports
References	Available upon request

FIGURE 10-1 A Sample Résumé

July 16, 2010

Suzanne Anderson, RDH
55 Hilltop Avenue
Riverview, California
(101) 555-0101
e-mail: sanderson@ internet.net

Dear Dr. Wells:

Enclosed you will find my résumé submitted in response to the position to the dental hygiene position advertised. My current goals include participating in patient education and promotion of optimal oral health while working in an atmosphere that provides a free exchange of ideas. I am experienced in many new aspects of dental technology, including digital radiography and intraoral cameras. Improving oral health care in patients is a priority, and I am well educated in many products that enhance home care therapies.

I am confident that upon review of my résumé, you will find I possess the skills necessary to enhance your dental team. In addition, I hope to provide organizational skills and extensive patient education to your practice. I look forward to meeting you and your staff at your earliest convenience. You may contact me at the address listed above.

Thank you for your consideration.

Sincerely,

Suzanne Anderson, RDH

FIGURE 10-2   A Sample Cover Letter

specific office, the cover letter should mention the individual who made the referral. It is a good idea to individualize each letter to the dentist or practice in which you are applying.

Cover letters allow you to introduce yourself. The letter may include identifying the practice's need for a certain quality or skill while pointing out that you may be the one to meet that need. Avoid replicating information that is found in the résumé itself. Cover letters are brief and may consist of one to three paragraphs. The first paragraph should state the reason for submitting the résumé for the position. You may also want to mention how you learned of the position. The second paragraph should explain the reason(s) for your interest in working with this practice and point out why you are the person for the position. The third paragraph can suggest meeting the employer in person and provide information on your availability or flexibility regarding the employer's schedule. Be sure to mention that there will be a follow-up on this communication. Finally, thank the employer for the opportunity and for his or her time in reviewing the résumé.

Post-Interview Acknowledgments

After interviewing with potential employers, sending a note of gratitude (see Figure 10-3) is considered courteous and is appreciated by employers and staff members who may have been involved in the interview process. This is also seen as a good marketing tool. The dental hygienist has acknowledged the time spent by the employer and reminded him or her of the meeting. It is also a great opportunity to market your skills and refresh the employer's memory on the

Dear Dr. Wells,

I appreciated having the opportunity to meet with you and your staff. I also appreciate the information you provided regarding your philosophy for dental care. I am greatly interested in working with you and your patients and feel I meet the qualifications you seek in a dental hygienist.

Sincerely,

Suzanne Anderson, RDH

FIGURE 10-3   A Sample Thank-you Letter

interview. Thank-you letters can be formal or simple. Specific points to consider for thank-you letters include the following:

- Be brief
- Restate your interest in the position
- Can be used as the follow-up contact
- Restate your qualifications

BEGINNING THE NEW JOB

Once the interviews have ended and the job offer is accepted, there are new aspects of employment and working in the dental hygiene profession that new practitioners will want to be informed of. For example, policy manuals, probationary periods, and compensation types are items not usually discussed during interviews. Additionally, many seasoned dental hygienists have indicated that negotiating skills would have helped them many times when it came to benefits.

Once the decision has been made to accept a position, the new dental hygienist will want to be prepared for the next phase of beginning the new job. Most new positions come with the understanding that a probationary period exists. This means that for a designated time (30 to 90 days), the new employee can leave the job at any time without stating a specific reason. During the probationary period, the employer also has the opportunity to terminate the agreement at any time. Most often, this period allows the employer to withhold benefits (if applicable) until both parties agree that the employment relationship will be extended indefinitely.

Compensation

Compensation is something that most new graduates look forward to as a dental hygienist. It is no secret that the compensation rate is attractive. However, there are many ways to be compensated as a dental hygienist. Salaries will vary all over the country and within the state where you reside. Currently, salary ranges can be found by contacting your local or state dental hygiene association. Some of the ways the practitioner can be compensated are found in Table 10-1. There are likely other ways to be compensated as a dental hygienist; however, these examples will give the new employee something to consider based on the type of practice. However you choose to be compensated, be very clear on the terms of the agreement. The bottom line is to be paid what you are worth. Many articles about compensation can be found in dental hygiene publications and professional organizations offer plentiful resources.

TABLE 10-1   Examples of Compensation for the Dental Hygienist

Type of Compensation	Description
Daily	The dental hygienist is paid a flat rate regardless of how much production is gained or the number of patients seen that day.
Base pay with commission	This means the practitioner will receive a base amount no matter what happens with scheduling. Any amount produced by the clinician over the base rate will be the amount of compensation for that day. For example, the base rate might be $200. Depending on the type of procedures scheduled, the production may have amounted to $950 for the day. If the commission is 40% of anything over the $200, the compensation for that day amounts to $300. This is the amount paid to the dental hygienist. Thus, the daily pay rate will vary.
Hourly	Hourly is based on a flat rate for the number of hours worked.
Commission only	This means that the dental hygienist has agreed to work for a certain commission or percentage of fees charged for services. Thus, no matter how many patients are seen or the type of treatment given, the daily rate is based on total production each day.
Commission on procedures	This is based on certain procedures being compensated over the agreed salary, whether it's a daily rate or not. For example, if the clinician performs four root planing cases in a day, the compensation is extra based on the agreement with the employer. Perhaps the dental hygienist negotiated an extra $30 per case. If the daily rate for compensation was $250, another $120 would be received for that day.

ANNUAL RAISES   Another aspect of compensation is an annual salary increase. More often than not, the dental hygienist is not included in annual increases because of the amount he or she is already paid. However, is this fair to any employee? This is an issue you may not be comfortable addressing at the start of a new job, but it is important to find out how the practice handles salary increases for its staff members. By addressing the question early, the professional dental hygienist can learn how to approach the subject in a timely manner. Most employers will not bring the subject up on a regular basis, so the employee must act in his or her own interest. According to a 2002 forecast by the U.S. Department of Labor, the number of dental hygienists is expected to increase 79% through 2012. The number of new programs opening on an annual basis indicates this growth.

OTHER CONSIDERATIONS   Many practices offer **merit** raises, which are based on the employee's performance and skills. Merit raises can occur annually or at the discretion of the employer. **Cost-of-living** raises may not be provided in many practices. These increases would also occur annually. They are based on the average cost it takes to maintain a standard of living (e.g., food, clothing, and medical expenses). Salary increases is a topic that any new employee will want to fully understand. Any time a salary increase is indicated and requested, be prepared to justify the increase.

Justification may include increased production in the dental hygiene department, broader responsibilities in the department, or the simple fact that you have been employed in the same office for several years. Some employers may use the cost of living index as a guide for salary increases. If increases are not provided for the dental hygienist, it can be something to negotiate at different points in your association with any practice.

Benefits

Benefits are likely the most important area for the dental hygienist to consider when seeking a position. As you may already know from many conversations with licensed practitioners and your instructors, **benefits** can be difficult to find for the dental hygienist. This is one area where many have voiced the need for negotiating tips so that some benefits are realized during their careers. Although there are dental hygiene positions that provide full benefits, such as those in education, public health, corporate environments, and some private-practice positions, these benefits are provided for full-time employment. Full time is generally defined as at least 32 hours per week. As mentioned, most dental hygienists prefer to work part time. A good benefit package may cost the employer approximately 20% of the employee's salary. Depending on the size of the practice, benefits can be expensive to the practice. Keep in mind that most dental practices are small businesses.

Major Benefit Components

Although benefits can vary widely, the major components will include the following:

Medical and dental	Sick days and well days/family leave	Holidays
Continuing education	Bonus incentives / Profit sharing	Retirement plans

HOLIDAYS   For many dental hygienists, the holidays can require advanced planning. Many practices choose to take several days off during the holidays. Legal holidays typically fall on Monday throughout the year. Be sure to ask what the normal practice for the office is during these times. For hygienists unable to take the same amount of time off, working as a substitute or temporary can alleviate loss of income during holidays. Other benefits, such as medical and dental, are more difficult but are available depending on the type of dental hygiene environment one chooses to be employed in.

COST OF BENEFITS   How would this break down from an employer's perspective? Using an example from *RDH* magazine, a benefit package based on an annual salary of $30,000 may look like that presented in Table 10-2. Since benefits vary from region to region and on an individual

TABLE 10-2   Sample Benefits Package

Benefit	Cost to Employer
2 weeks of vacation per year	$723.20 (based on $9.04/per hour × 80 hours)
5 sick days per year	$45.20
Health insurance (annual)	$2,000–$3,000 for single persons/$6,000–$7,200 for families
Continuing education	$400
Uniform allowance	$50/month
Free dental care	$220 (this may only cover a lab fee)
Bonus—production	$219/month
Total package	**$4,207.40 minimum per employee**

Source: Bureau of Labor Statistics, 2010.

basis; this represents only a sample of what the employer must spend to provide a package to employees. Dental hygienists can use this information to their advantage, as many will be able to negotiate portions of a benefit package and enhance their compensation. *RDH* magazine publishes the annual "Salary and Benefits Survey." For more information on salary ranges and benefits offered to dental hygienists, research *RDH* magazine, through their website.

Case Study Follow-up #2

After going through the section on benefits, prioritize some of the benefits based on needs of the staff members and determine which benefits the staff might be willing to decrease or eliminate.

Negotiating

What will it take to incorporate negotiating skills in preparation for interviews and annual **evaluations**? Negotiating is not in the comfort zone for many individuals. Since the majority of dental hygienists are women, it becomes an aspect that even fewer are comfortable in implementing. Negotiating often has more to do with being a newcomer and having no leverage than with being a woman. Julie Nierenberg, coauthor of *Women and the Art of Negotiation* (1999), states that "one of the most overlooked features of negotiating successfully is trying to figure everything from the other point of view. We're so stuck in our own point of view that we don't stop to consider, how will they look at all of this?" Therefore, to gain any aspect of benefits, the big picture is what each new employee must keep in mind. Numerous books and Internet resources are available to those who seek more information about negotiating skills (key word: "negotiating skills"). However, some of the basics listed in Box 10-4 can be provided in order for students and new graduates to familiarize themselves with the process.

Other Negotiating Considerations

Approach is another aspect of negotiating that requires attention. During the interview, keep in mind that the office wants to hire you. As health care providers, both parties share the same goal. Flexibility must be exercised, and each person must remain honest and fair. If benefit requests are not met on the first attempt, inquire as to when they can be revisited. If the practice is observant of annual employee evaluations, the next benefit on the list can be discussed at that time. The most important aspect to remember is that you must be willing to walk away. Even as a new graduate and a new employee, you have many positions available to you.

To be successful at negotiating benefits, whether it is one benefit or an entire package, walking away is something to be prepared for. When negotiating benefits, keep in mind what may seem as minor items. For example, if you accept a position out of your immediate community and commuting is required, how about negotiating for gas expense? It may not take into account the wear and tear on your vehicle, but it will assist in the cost of fuel. Over time, this expense adds up. This is the first step in negotiating benefits.

As experience is gained, the dental hygienist becomes more in tune to what he or she seeks in a benefits package. If benefits are never an option for the dental hygienist, taking small steps is the next-best option.

BOX 10-4

Negotiating Basics

Your Negotiation

- No two experiences are alike because of the differences in your needs, the market, and where you are in your career.
- Make a list of your needs (financial, working days, hours, etc.). This will help you stay focused during the interview and bring out the things you are looking for in your employment agreement.

Do Your Research

- Will the employer negotiate? Do you know others who work in the same office? If so, discuss the dentists' flexibility in meeting the needs of employees.
- Who is the decision maker? It is not always the dentist-it could be the wife, or a practice management consultant. Whom will you be interviewed by? This will make a difference in your negotiation and you may have to be brought back for more interviews.

Know Your Priorities

- Is it salary, benefits, or bonuses? New graduates report getting offers for lower salaries because they are "new." Will this be acceptable for your needs? If not, perhaps this is not the practice for you. In order to meet your needs, be sure to know what areas you are willing to be flexible and in what areas you must stay firm.

Stay Focused on Long-Term Goals

- Will trade-offs occur? In order to get hired, are you giving up on one or more of your needs? Will they be met at a later date? You are the only one who can determine which terms are acceptable.
- Be ready to justify your needs and requirements. If one of your needs includes day care for young children, be sure to inform the employer of limits to your working hours. If you are seeking a certain salary level, your employer needs to know in advance so that you both work together to meet that mark.
- Compare your career or job to others that include benefits. If you need or want health benefits, discuss and negotiate terms that work for both you and your employer.

Source: Kimberly Wandel, *Wisdom Technologies*

Case Study Follow-up #3

The other staff members have elected you to present and negotiate a new benefit package with the dentist. Outline the strategy you will take based on the negotiating basics presented in Box 10-4.

Employment Contracts

Some practices extend an employment contract to their employees. This type of contract can be advantageous to both the employer and the employee because it helps eliminate possible misunderstandings of expectations on both sides. Employment contracts will have numerous categories, and you should carefully review the contract if presented by the employer. These contracts are another area for negotiation. The dental hygienist can also develop and present a contract as they are not limited to employers in their creation.

Most employment contracts will cover topics such as the following:

Position and duties to be performed	Evaluation periods: 90 days, annually
Work schedule: Days/hours	Salary increase schedule/type of increase (e.g., cost of living/merit)
Compensation: Amount and how the compensation is calculated and paid	Fringe benefits (e.g., continuing education uniform)
Pay schedule: Weekly, semi-monthly	Vacations/holidays
Benefits and how they are deducted from a paycheck	Termination of employment methods/process

Policy Manuals

Office **policy manuals** are likely to be found in most practices. It is of benefit and good business practice for the office to have them on hand and to provide a copy for all staff members. They assist in decreasing misunderstandings about what the practice will provide to its staff members as well as expectations it has of employees. Policy manuals will range in complexity, again based on the size and scope of the practice. However, basic topics such as those identified in Box 10-5 will be found in all manuals.

Many categories in employment contracts and office policy manuals are similar. They are all designed to inform staff members of expectations and to decrease misunderstandings during employment with the practice.

Employee Evaluations

Evaluations are provided for staff members, typically on an annual basis, so that employees can be informed of their strong points and areas where improvement might be necessary and the employer and employee can discuss other aspects of the duties. Dental hygienists may not participate in an evaluation, but many feel this would benefit the professional working relationship. One reason dental hygienists may not be provided evaluations is because regular salary increases may not be included during employment. However, it gives both the dentist and the dental hygienist a chance to discuss philosophy and new programs that have entered the practice for the patient and to touch base on operations. During the interview process or shortly after beginning a new position, inquire as to the evaluation process in the office and ask to participate. It is an advantage for the professional to continuously provide information as well as participate in changes that occur in the office. Evaluations are one avenue that can be used by the dental hygienist.

BOX 10-5

Contents of Policy Manuals

Terms of employment (describes the type of employment offered)	General employment definitions/requirements	Work schedule
• Equal opportunity • At-will (termination can come from either party at any time for any reason), contracts • Sexual harassment policy • Risk management/safety procedures	• Full time/part time (defined) • Temporary (defined) • Waiting period determined prior to onset of benefits • License requirements/maintaining licensure	• Office hours • Individual work schedules • Who works when doctors are out of the office • Time cards/tardiness • Lunch breaks/breaks • Staff meetings

Compensation issues	Employee benefits	Dress and appearance
• Types of compensation • Flexible work arrangements • Overtime duties/compensation • Bonus pay/severance pay • Pay periods/salary advances • Performance evaluations • Job abandonment (termination without notice)	• Vacations/holidays • Sick time • Health insurance/dental benefits/ retirement plans • Continuing education • Workers' compensation • Jury duty • Leaves of absence • Bereavement leave • Pregnancy leave	• Personal hygiene • Hair • Nails • Jewelry • Gum chewing • Shoes • Uniform attire

Additional sections

Conduct during work/Personal business on company time/Office supplies/Confidentiality/Noncompetition clauses (competing for business from patients while at work). For example, many offices have lunch rooms or break rooms where staff and patients may leave merchandise catalogs and staff are able to purchase goods via mail order.

Summary

Job searching requires thoughtful planning. The availability of dental hygiene positions must be considered when initiating the search. Some find they begin by commuting to outlying areas, and some find they prefer to relocate to new communities. Working as a temporary can be a source of stable income as well as a flexible choice for employment. Interviews are done by employers and should also be conducted by the potential employee. Three key characteristics can be incorporated to assist in active participation of interviews: being proactive, looking at the end result, and the desire of a win-win outcome. Gaining employment may also consist of personality tests, employment testing, and numerous questions on professional and personal aspects. Working interviews can be advantageous for both the applicant and the employer, as they allow each person to work with the other to determine if their philosophies mesh. Résumés are necessary to promote skills and qualifications. Formats are easily available, and numerous other avenues are readily available to ensure a quality document. Résumés will contain specific sections with concise information for any potential employer to review easily. Typically, cover letters accompany all résumés, and sending a post-interview acknowledgment is another way to remind the employer of the meeting.

Compensation comes in many forms. The new graduate will want to carefully review what is being offered and how it will fit into his or her plan as a professional. Everything is negotiable, and incorporating some skills will assist in obtaining the overall goal as the career begins. Benefits are also negotiable, and there are some dental hygiene positions that provide full benefits. Clinicians are encouraged to expand and seek positions that enhance the clinical aspect of their careers. Policy manuals are found in nearly all practices and are provided to inform staff members of the benefits provided as well as to define each person's duties. They also define the parameters for leaves of absence and workers' compensation.

Critical Thinking

1. In this group exercise, one group member is seeking employment in one of the environments listed below. Create a list of questions that will be used during an interview with the potential employer. Be sure to design questions that target the practice environment chosen. In addition, a second group member can prepare questions as if he or she were the employer. At the end of the exercise, role-play an interview session.
   a. General practice
   b. Periodontal practice
   c. Pedodontic practice
   d. Community dental clinic
   e. Federal Native American reservation
   f. Hospital dental provider (providing dental hygiene services to the developmentally disabled)

2. Create a résumé that you will use when you begin seeking employment. Be sure to include all sections pertinent to your experience and education as well as references. Be sure to create a cover letter and a post-interview acknowledgment.

3. As a dental hygienist in a new practice, you have been asked to create a section of the policy manual that will address all dental hygienists employed by the practice. Provide the information required for the policy manual. Be sure to address working hours and days, compensation methods, job descriptions, and benefits that will apply.

4. Identify and briefly explain the types of salary increases that may occur in the dental practice.

5. Organize a job fair with local dentists to gain interview experience.

CHAPTER 11

Planning for the Future and Career Longevity

OBJECTIVES

After reading the material in this chapter, you will be able to

- Describe the differences between *stocks, mutual funds*, and *IRAs*.
- Explain the meaning of *portfolio*.
- Describe *CD investments*.
- Explain *liability insurance*.
- Explain *disability insurance*.
- Identify the need for *self-care* and *physical health*.
- Describe the benefits of *professional membership*.

KEY TERMS

Compounding interest	Life insurance	Online trading
Disability	Malpractice	Portfolio
Liability	Net worth	

INTRODUCTION

As students graduate and enter a field of flexible working schedules and financial independence, getting a head start on retirement through wise investment strategies is the next step in continuing education. Federal retirement vehicles such as social security benefits are constantly being reviewed and debated in the political arena each year. The Social Security program is funded through payroll deductions from those working in the United States. Upon retirement, Social Security is one source of income, yet it is very little compared to a dental hygiene salary. As the cost of living increases, so will the cost for those reaching retirement. New graduates (regardless of age) are recommended to begin an investment **portfolio** (a summary of all investments held) so that retirement includes financial security. Not only is retirement a good reason to invest, many dental hygienists will want to send their children to college, purchase a vacation home, or just be assured of financial security. Essentially, you want to invest in something that will assist in creating wealth to gain enough money for a comfortable retirement income.

Many dental hygiene practitioners will work in clinical practice for many years. There are numerous clinicians who have practiced for 20 years and more. After working as a dental hygienist for a while, some have found that the physical stress has begun to take a toll on their body. The neck, shoulder, lower back, and carpal tunnel areas contribute to career longevity. When these areas become stressed and damaged from repeated movement, the aging process, or both, a career as a dental hygienist becomes limited. In order to maintain systemic and physical health, the clinician has numerous options that can be incorporated into everyday living. This chapter will introduce common mechanisms for retirement planning and investing along with preventive practices to insure a long and productive career.

Case Study

You have been working with the same practice for 5 years. During that time the practice has grown substantially, and the dentist has started to provide some benefits based on the number of years staff members have been employed. As a single person, you would like to see retirement benefits included since most of the staff members have no retirement plan through a spouse. Your annual performance evaluation is scheduled for next week, so you decide to present your idea to the dentist.

As you read this chapter, consider the following: Use the Internet to research retirement plans using these keywords: Roth IRA, traditional IRA, and 401(k). Which of these investment plans would benefit both the practice and the employer?

THE BASICS OF INVESTING

When considering investments or savings accounts, be sure to spend some time investigating the returns given on the initial investment. For example, most banking institutions pay only 1% to 2% (2010 rates) interest/return per year on a regular savings account. Therefore, if $2,000 is placed in the account and nothing is added for the year, the return would range from $60 to $100—not much for hard-earned dollars. However, if that same $2,000 was placed into a retirement plan and $1,000 was added each year, averaging 9% compound interest over 30 years, the investment would be worth $175,110 (http:www.moneychimp.com, 2010).

However, not all investments will be successful. Those who choose higher risk investments are actually investing in the stock market. So, on any given day, if the stock market (Dow Jones or Nasdaq) goes down in value, the money invested decreases. Given this information, it is wise to find an investment broker who will assist in the type of retirement plan that will achieve the goals desired, no matter what you save for.

DETERMINE INVESTMENT GOALS   Financial planning means looking at your personal situation, outlining goals, and developing an action plan that will achieve them (see Box 11-1). By doing so, you remain focused on the success of the outcome. When you initiate an investment plan, most financial firms will take time to outline some basic steps:

BOX 11-1

Basic Planning Considerations

- Identify, prioritize, and quantify financial goals and objectives. Begin by listing goals you want to accomplish: an individual retirement plan, a college fund, and so on.
- Summarize personal data and records so that they are easy to follow. Develop a file that includes the type of investments owned and frequently update it to display **net worth** (amount of money remaining after all debts are paid).
- Compare goals to investments. Be sure that your investments are working to their best ability, that the interest rate is still competitive, and that the investment is still viable.
- Develop a savings and investment plan that is specific to your needs. It may include mutual funds, stocks, and certificates of deposit (CDs).
- Monitor progress on a regular basis.

There are numerous avenues available for investors. It is easy to get started while becoming more familiar with the different markets. Table 11-1 summarizes some of these avenues.

Investment Vehicles

Now that the basics of investing avenues have been outlined, what is the next step? First, decide what type of investments you are willing to explore. There are risks in any investment.

HIGH-RISK INVESTMENTS In the high-risk category are stocks. During the end of the 20th century and beyond, technology stocks were a hot commodity—volatile to say the least, but many young investors became millionaires practically overnight. However, if retirement is the main objective, stocks could be too risky. In 2008 the stock market plummeted, nearly matching the fall it took during the Great Depression. When investing in high-risk vehicles, be aware that the investment will rise and fall with fluctuations in the stock market.

MEDIUM-RISK INVESTMENTS Mutual funds are medium-risk investments. A mutual fund is a collection of stocks, bonds, or other securities owned by a large group of often small investors. This is a way to invest in many companies at one time. When using mutual funds as a retirement vehicle, you are investing in multiple types of companies along with thousands of other investors. This allows pooled money to gain interest at a faster rate. Although the return on investment will not be as high as on stocks, it is a safer, more conservative mechanism to achieve the targeted goal. Many mutual funds will provide a return of 11% to over 20% per year.

IRAS Independent retirement accounts (IRAs) are another medium- to low-risk area where the investment is conservative. They also provide a tax break (depending on the IRAs chosen) with regular annual deposits by the investor. Some IRAs allow the investor to place $2,500 to $4,500 each year, which is considered tax deferred. Tax will not be imposed on these funds

TABLE 11-1 Investment Vehicles	
Investment method	**Description**
Short-term investments	
Savings accounts	Banking institutions. Offering mainly 2% to 4% per year on the investment.
Money market funds	Specialized form of mutual funds. Usually pay better interest rates than savings accounts but lower than CDs.
CDs	Specialized deposits made at a bank or other financial institution. Interest rates are higher and may vary depending on the length of the deposit. CDs mature and can be reinvested or cashed with the accumulated interest.
Long-term investments	
Bonds	Available in various forms. Are known as "fixed-income" securities because they generate a fixed income each year. Similar to CDs, but they are issued by a government agency.
Stock	A "share" of stock represents a share of ownership in a company. When the value of the company changes, the value of the stock changes.
Mutual funds	Includes stocks, bonds, and other vehicles. Mutual funds are a collection of investments in one place. Interest rates fluctuate, yet investments can earn over 30% per year.
Retirement plans	
IRA	Allows income to be placed into a tax-deferred fund (you do not pay taxes on the income until it is withdrawn).
Roth IRA	A new plan that offers total exemption from federal taxes on withdrawal. No tax advantages are offered up front, however (cannot be deducted from yearly income taxes). There are income restrictions ($95,000/single; $150,000/married).
401(k)	Offered by employers. Usually, the employer matches the funds invested by the employee (if employee invests 10% of salary per month, the employer contributes 10%).
Retirement plans	
403(b)	Used in nonprofit organizations similar to the 401(k) plan (local and state governments).
Keogh	Specialty IRA. It doubles as a pension plan for self-employed persons. It is limited to $30,000 per year.
Simplified employee pension (SEP) plan	Special kind of Keogh IRA created for small businesses. Employees and employers make contributions.

until withdrawn upon retirement. If funds are withdrawn prior to retirement, the investor has to pay taxes along with a 10% penalty. IRAs are proven vehicles that will help in meeting that retirement goal.

CERTIFICATES OF DEPOSIT   In the low-risk category are certificates of deposit (CDs) and bank saving accounts. They are designed to be short or medium-term investments. CDs can have a maturity period of 6 months, 1 year, and 2 years. The investor agrees to leave the money in the

CDs for a period. Low interest rates of 3% to 4% are generally associated with CDs and savings accounts. Early withdrawal of these funds will also result in a penalty. Typically, these types of vehicles will not be an advantage to build a large retirement fund unless you are able to make significant deposits each month and begin at an early age.

Earned Interest

There are several types of earned interest when money is put into an investment fund or savings account. Here are a few examples:

Compounding interest is an advantage if you are attentive to how it works. Compounding interest adds to the initial investment as a result of interest rate and the amount of time the funds remain untouched. When interest is added to the principal investment, it too earns interest so the original amount of money gets larger. The more money you can put into a savings account without withdrawing it, the faster your account grows because of interest gained year after year. Be sure to ask an investment broker what avenues will gain the best compound interest based on the type of investments you choose for your portfolio. Some financial investments require a specific amount to open an account, and many may require an annual administrative fee. No matter what avenue is selected to begin a retirement portfolio, it will require the expertise of a broker to explain how many investments work. Take the time to investigate how a retirement plan will work best for you.

Case Study Follow-up #1

Using Table 11-1, determine what type of IRA would most benefit employees. Would your choice benefit the employer as well? If not, which retirement plan would be better?

Investment Brokers

What do investment brokers do? Essentially, they are salespersons. They will be the ones to purchase stocks or mutual funds as requested or recommended by you. Brokers are paid on commission, salary, or both. No matter their compensation, they are experts in investing and building a portfolio to suit your needs. Recently, both novice and experienced investors have begun to participate in **online trading**. This type of investing requires watching and constant monitoring of the stock market. There are numerous investment firms that have online trading available for their clients. However, this is not recommended unless you have the time to monitor your investments and have extensive knowledge of online trading.

SPEND MONEY WISELY

One of the golden rules for investing in a savings mechanism is to "pay yourself first." Many individuals are credit card poor. This means that hard-earned dollars are spent trying to pay down credit card balances every month. However, if the interest rate on the card is 18% to 23% (which is the average), making that debt disappear will take years. While paying the bills, add one more: yourself. In fact, it should be the first bill paid every month. After all, if the money is invested today, it begins to work tomorrow. The interest on that credit card does not. Many investment experts suggest that a percentage of income be identified early so that regardless of gross or net salary, a predetermined amount has been set aside each month. For those who participate in an employer-paid retirement plan, like a 401(k), 8% may be the amount invested by the employee and matched by the employer. Setting a goal of 10% each month will assist in reaching financial goals earlier. In addition, avoid pitfalls that occur every day to those who want to invest and never seem to accomplish the task:

- Do nothing.
- Start late (better late than never, though).
- Paying down the credit card (better to pay yourself).
- Turn down the retirement plan offered by an employer.

Although each individual or family will have to decide on what is best for them, it is wise to put away as much as possible. This will ensure a stable financial future.

INSURANCE COVERAGE FOR DENTAL HYGIENISTS

Along with retirement planning and investments, graduates and practicing professionals are wise to protect themselves by insuring their skills and protecting themselves from possible lawsuits. Life insurance, disability, and liability are three key policies recommended for all practitioners.

Liability Coverage

During dental hygiene education, many students protect themselves from possible lawsuits by purchasing **liability** insurance. Once licensed, dental hygienists typically continue with this coverage. Liability coverage is essentially **malpractice** insurance. It protects the clinician against financial loss should he or she be named in a negligence, technical battery, or other lawsuit. Policies can vary among carriers, and the practitioner will want to educate himself or herself on what will be covered in the policy. Benefits are limited and will vary from company to company. For example, an average policy for a dental hygienist may cover up to $3 million per lifetime, with $1 million paid per year per incident as the maximum benefit. The annual premium for such a policy may range from $70 to $90. As a member of your professional organization, this type of coverage is available at a group rate.

Disability Coverage Disability

Disability insurance will assist the professional with monthly income if unable to work for an extended period. Suppose the dental hygienist breaks a wrist while skiing or has complications after childbirth and cannot return to work as planned. Disability insurance will provide a certain amount of income (approximately 50% of monthly compensation) so that financial obligations can be met. This may help keep bankruptcy in the wings. Additionally, many dental hygienists have been placed on permanent disability because of severe latex allergies and spinal stress disorders due to long-term clinical practice. When this occurs, it prevents the professional from working in a clinical setting, but there are many other positions that can be held by a dental hygienist. Disability premiums range from carrier to carrier and through professional membership, group rates can be obtained.

Many studies are done regarding statistics on musculoskeletal disorders among dental health care workers. Smith and Cockrell (2009) studied a group of dental hygiene students and found that 62.3% reported neck problems, 58% reported lower back problems, and 48.4% reported stress in the shoulder regions. Because of the high incidence of carpal tunnel syndrome and cumulative stress disorders, many private carriers do not consider the dental hygienist (as they are at a higher risk). Finding coverage will require some investigation on the part of the practitioner. Many policies require higher premiums or waiting periods before benefits begin, and some may have a threshold on benefits paid over a certain amount of time. Be sure to spend some time with the insurance agent to gain a complete understanding of what the policy entails and to be sure it is right for your lifestyle and the way you practice. Many states provide disability insurance based on earnings over the past 9 months. However, the benefits are far less than what a good disability policy can provide. Dental hygiene salaries can be substantial. State disability will not be adequate should you be out of work for an extended period.

Life Insurance Coverage

Life insurance is another consideration for many practitioners with families. In case of unforeseen tragedy, plan wisely as your family may suffer with unpaid debts and taxes. Life insurance is the farthest thing from the minds of graduates who begin their careers at a young age. No matter your age, life insurance is something to initiate at the start of a new career. Premiums for life insurance will depend on age. Typically, mature people pay a higher premium. However, by holding a life insurance policy, your family will be financially stable should their financial support unexpectedly cease.

Term or Whole-Life Policies

Life insurance policies also vary. There is term life and cash value. Term life insurance provides death protection for a stated period, or term. Term life insurance is perhaps the simplest form of life insurance. It was developed to provide temporary life insurance protection on a limited budget. Since term insurance can be purchased in large amounts for a relatively small initial premium, it is well suited for short-range goals such as life insurance coverage to pay off a loan, or providing extra life insurance protection during the child-raising years (State Farm Insurance Company, 2010). A savings account can be developed with a term insurance policy and consulting your insurance agent is recommended for more complete information.

Cash value, or *whole life*, is a combination of insurance coverage and a savings account. Whole life is permanent life insurance protection that protects your family or business no matter what lies ahead, from the day you purchase the policy until you die, as long as you pay the premiums when due (New York Life, 2010). The interest rate on a whole-life policy is typically low compared to other investment options. When investigating the type of life insurance policy right for you and your family, be sure to analyze the options.

CONSIDER BENEFIT OPTIONS   Many dental hygienists find they must provide their own health insurance once they begin practice. Unless the practitioner negotiates benefits with the employer, the entire cost falls to the clinician. Many states have plans similar to those of Blue Cross or Blue Shield available for consumer purchase. Simply making a phone call will provide necessary information to obtain an individual or family policy. Furthermore, some states have health maintenance organizations (HMOs) that may offer their coverage and services to individuals or families who are not employed with a large company. Any insurance company will let you know what type of insurance plans it provides. Not all carriers will provide everything the dental hygienist may need or desire. Thus, you may be referred to other insurance carriers. Be prepared to spend some time finding the carrier and policies designed for you.

PROFESSIONAL MEMBERSHIP

Many dental hygiene programs offer or require students to join the Student Chapter of the American Dental Hygienists' Association. Upon graduation and licensure, active membership in the professional organization becomes an advantage in many ways. First, insurance companies offer group rates to organizations. Many find that this benefit suits their financial plan since many premiums are expensive. The American Dental Hygienists' Association (ADHA) offers many types of insurance coverage to its members. In addition to disability, liability, life, and supplemental medical, home, and auto insurance can also be purchased through the ADHA. However, the policy limitations may differ from a private carrier. The most common variations are in the length of benefits, the maximum of benefits, the deductible, and the waiting period. Again, it is worthwhile to compare policies. For more information on insurance benefits through ADHA, visit the website at www.adha.org.

MEMBER BENEFITS   Insurance is only one benefit of membership, and it is a tangible benefit. Intangible benefits are more numerous and may be of more value than tangible benefits. Undoubtedly, dental hygiene students have been introduced to their professional organization at some level: national, state, or local. Annual membership fees are relatively inexpensive for the many benefits provided: approximately the compensation received for one day's work—easy enough to come by and are also tax deductible. Intangible benefits include networking with other professionals, participating in legislative issues, mentoring, representing the local component to the national organization, educational support, continuing education, and research avenues.

Patient Perspective

From the consumer's perspective, membership in a professional organization indicates that the practitioner maintains a high level of knowledge for new trends in patient care. When perusing the telephone directory in any community, one observes that physicians and dentists identify their degrees and any fellowships held in their field of education or practice by the letters attached to the name. This need not be any different for the licensed dental hygienist. Identification of membership in the ADHA, its state, and local components tells the patient that you are involved and take interest in your profession. Many practitioners believe they owe it to their patients to be a member in their professional associations. The benefits are numerous, both tangible and intangible. It is wise for new licentiates to maintain their membership while maintaining their license.

SELF-CARE

As learned in dental hygiene programs, the practice of ergonomics will be essential to the longevity of one's career. Protecting skeletal muscles and avoiding carpal tunnel problems, are two important aspects of dental hygiene practice to keep in mind in order to sustain overall physical health.

Cumulative Trauma Disorders

Cumulative trauma disorder (CTD) is defined as musculoskeletal disorders that can result from the body's inability to heal itself from the long-term effects of repetitive motion, exposure to vibration, and mechanical stress. According to the U.S. Bureau of Labor Statistics,

CTD is the fastest-growing occupational disorder. A study done by Anton, Rosecrance, Merlino, and Cook (2002), resulted in 93% of the participants (N = 95), reporting at least one CTD. The dental hygiene profession remains among the top 10 occupations for CTD. Although many aspects of dental hygiene have seen modification to reduce stress disorders by practicing ergonomics, students and practitioners will want to remain active and healthy to increase career longevity. No longer do clinicians grasp small-diameter instruments; there is a diverse selection of handles that make it easier for the clinician to decrease muscle fatigue in the hands and wrists. Operator chairs are now ergonomically designed to provide better lower-back support and a place to rest the forearm. Ultrasonic units and slow-speed hand pieces have been designed specifically to decrease the weight and vibrations placed on the practitioner's arms and wrists.

ERGONOMICS IN PRACTICE   Body positioning in relation to the patient plays an important part in posture while scaling and root planing all day long. Exercise is a priority for those who want to ensure the length of their careers. Clinicians should avoid slouching over the patient for direct vision and should work more with the mirror, eliminating the stress placed on the spine. Many students tend to cross their ankles or legs while working in the seven o'clock position. This puts stress on the spine and may create muscle fatigue on the lower back, as the body must lean slightly to maintain an upright position. Patients are willing to comply so that the clinician gains better access. Ask the patient to turn his or her head, tilt upward, tilt downward, or whatever it takes to decrease the stress on your body. Some patients are not able to comply because of their own medical or physical condition. However, this is not likely to happen every day in private practice unless the practitioner is employed with a facility caring for such patients. For these patients, practitioners will have to compensate their positioning for the patient. Good preventive practice will be to perform wrist and body stretches throughout the day.

BOX 11-2

Features for Dental Operatories

   1. The size of the room: Will you have enough space to work in the twelve o'clock position without bumping into cabinets? Be sure the range of movement around the patient chair provides enough access that good body mechanics can continue.

   2. Lighting: Many older practices may not have adequate lighting in the room or in the overhead light for the patient. This may cause increased stress on vision and body mechanics, as the clinician may constantly have to lean over or get closer to the oral cavity to see the working area adequately.

   3. Access to equipment and supplies: Pay attention to the location of the ultrasonic unit and supplies that are in the workspace. Are they located within easy reach, or are they in a location that will require excessive stretching during the treatment period? If the clinician has to continuously reach for items needed during treatment, body mechanics tend to be stressed. Over a long period(weeks, months, or years), this stress may cause undue stress disorders that could require medical attention.

Dental Operatories

Once you have graduated and are seeking employment, it will be beneficial to discuss ergonomics with potential employers. Many seasoned practices are in buildings that have been standing for over 30 years. Clinic operatory space was not designed to allow much room around the dental chair so that assistants and dentists could have supplies easily accessible (see Box 11-2). When touring dental offices during interviews, ask to see the room where you may be working. Some specifics to look for include the following:

Healthy Lifestyle

In order to increase career longevity, the dental hygienist must place his or her health first. This includes diet and exercise. A balanced diet full of nutritious foods will help you avoid the common cold, influenza, and other seasonal, communicable diseases that occur in patients seen every day all year long. Water consumption remains the number one objective in the best of diets. Keep the body hydrated, and consume fruits and vegetables more frequently than starchy items. Limit saturated fats and sugars. By doing so, body weight and body fat can be managed, and energy levels will increase. A balanced diet can help protect against harmful systemic diseases.

Exercise plays an important role in maintaining a healthy posture through strengthening the muscles that surround the skeletal system. For many, membership in a health club is the only thing that will motivate them to exercise. For others, taking advantage of the outdoors through various activities keeps them active. The American College of Sports Medicine recommends that exercise be done at least 30 minutes every day. Other sources may recommend four or five times per week. Exercise comes in various forms; however, just walking will provide activity and improved health. An activity plan may also require some time management in order to fit it into a busy schedule. Lunch breaks are a great opportunity to walk for 30 minutes. Participating in organized functions like walk-a-thons and races is another way to spend some time outside those operatory walls.

No matter the choice of activity to incorporate into your lifestyle, the benefits will be seen in a variety of ways:

- Weight loss/increased muscle tone
- Increased energy/healthier food choices
- Decreased depression/increased social interaction
- Decreased illness

By making subtle changes in lifestyle, many practitioners will realize career longevity. Furthermore, many of the CTDs are decreased, thus decreasing the possibility of surgical procedures.

Therapeutic Considerations

Another preventive measure for muscle and skeletal fatigue is massage therapy. This may be one of the most popular and successful avenues in the prevention of stress disorders. Massage therapy on a regular basis aids not only in relaxing tight muscles around the skeletal system but also in relaxing the mind. It allows the practitioner some quiet time that helps alleviate the mental and physical stresses of dental hygiene procedures. Many physicians advocate the value of including massage therapy in your preventive care routine. There are dental practices that have begun to include a massage therapist in their benefits for employees. The dentist will have the massage therapist visit the practice once a month and provide 15-minute sessions to employees. This assists in the overall wellness of staff members. Massage therapy can be scheduled as easily as a hair appointment and is a relatively inexpensive preventive measure that can add to career longevity. Millions of dollars are lost annually by dental practitioners because of CTDs and related pain. Take proactive measures to ensure that it does not happen to you or your family.

For those who are experiencing some kind of CTD or other condition, you are not alone. There are many who currently experience some kind of pain. Myofacial pain, myalgia, carpal tunnel, and neck and shoulder problems are among a few. Musculoskeletal disorders have become so prevalent that many questions can be answered through Internet medical sites such as WebMD (www.webmd.com). Additionally, articles can be found in dental hygiene journals. These resources and related sites may provide answers to questions on preventing cumulative stress disorders.

No matter the type of exercise or activity you choose, a balanced diet is essential for a healthy lifestyle. Numerous preventive measures must be employed, and the dental hygienist will want to make a concerted effort to lengthen the life of his or her chosen profession. The cost of a dental hygiene education can be abruptly interrupted without the proper fitness routine. Each professional will want to take the time to organize his or her career to benefit from the effort put into reaching one's educational and career goals. The key to career longevity is to prevent cumulative stress disorders.

Summary

Upon graduation, financial planning is the first step to ensure that retirement goals are realized. Developing financial goals and seeking expert advice will assist in outlining a financial plan best suited to your specific needs. A diverse portfolio is one of the best ways to increase self-wealth. There are numerous avenues available for investments, and it will take some research to select the best investments to meet your retirement goals. Investments range from high risk to low risk. Each individual and family will want to select investments wisely. Insurance coverage for dental hygienists is recommended. Disability insurance provides benefits if you are unable to work because of long-term illness, medical complications, or accident. Liability or malpractice insurance provides benefits in the event of lawsuits in which the dental hygienist is named. There are limitations on the amount of benefits provided per year and per lifetime. Life insurance will provide for those family members who remain in the event of an untimely death. Premiums for all types of insurance policies vary, as do the companies that offer them. Membership in your professional organization will assist in tangible and intangible benefits. Career longevity will depend on how well the practitioner maintains his or her health. Avoidance of musculoskeletal disorders must be a priority if the dental hygienist plans on a long professional career. Preventive measures include ergonomically designed instruments and equipment as well as a balanced diet and regular exercise.

Critical Thinking

1. Describe the differences between a stock and a mutual fund.
2. Why are mutual funds a better investment than a CD from your local bank?
3. What is the meaning and intent of a diverse portfolio?
4. Obtain a copy of the local newspaper and locate the stock report. Select five companies and find out how much a share costs to purchase. After three days, locate the same five companies to see the change in value. For example, locate Microsoft, General Motors, Wal-Mart, Amazon.com, and Home Depot.
5. Explain why the dental hygienist will want to consider purchasing disability insurance.
6. List some of the benefits of a healthy lifestyle.
7. Visit the ADHA's website and research tangible and intangible benefits. Share your thoughts about membership with classmates.

APPENDIX A

Internet Resources

Miles and Associates
http://www.dentalmanagementu.com/

American Academy of Pediatrics
http://www.aap.org

American Association of Retired People
http://www.aarp.org

American Dental Association
http://www.ada.org

American Dental Education Association
http://www.adea.org

American Dental Hygienists' Association
http://www.adha.org

Advanced Dental Education Institute
http://www.learndental.com/index.html

The Basics of Team Building
*http://www.teamtechnology.co.uk/tt/t-articl/
tb-basic.htm*

Belmont Report
http://www.hhs.gov/ohrp/belmontArchive.html

Bplans.com Business Plan Templates and Samples
http://www.bplans.com/sample_business_plans.cfm

Canadian Dental Hygienists Association
http://www.cdha.ca

Canadian HIV/AIDS Legal Network
http://www.aidslaw.ca

Centers for Disease Control
http://www.cdc.gov

Central Regional Dental Testing Service, Inc. (CRDTS)
http://www.crdts.org

"Characteristics of an Effective Team"
http://clce.gmu.edu/leadership/leadtips.html

Child Abuse Prevention Network™
http://www.child-abuse.com

Childhelp USA: Treatment and Prevention of Child Abuse
http://www.childhelpusa.org

Community–Campus Partnership for Health
(service learning)
http://www.ccph.info

Creative Job Search: Dress and Grooming for Job Success
http://www.mnworkforcecenter.org

Equal Employment Opportunity Commission (EEOC)
http://www.eeoc.gov

Health Canada
*http://www.hc-sc.gc.ca/english/care/romanow/
hcc0403.html*

Health Canada, Canada Health Act
http://www.hc-sc.gc.ca/index-eng.php

Health Care Financing Administration
http://www.hhs.gov/about/opdivs/hcfa.html

"How to Build a Team"
http://clce.gmu.edu/leadership/leadtips.html

How to Successfully Write and Negotiate a Contract,
Robbi Erickson
*http://www.googobits.com/articles/2667-how-to-
successfully-write-and-negotiate-a-contract.html*

Infection Control in Dental Health Care
*http://www.cdc.gov/mmwr/review/mmwrhtml/
rr5217al.htm*

Information and Knowledge for Optimal
Health (INFO) Project
http://www.infoforhealth.org

International Federation of Dental Hygienists
http://ifdh.org

Investing Basics
http://www.fool.com/investing/basics/index.aspx

The Leaders Institute
http://www.leadersinstitute.com

National Clearinghouse on Child Abuse and Neglect
and National Adoption Information Clearinghouse
*http://www.happinessonline.org/
LoveAndHelpChildren/p7.htm*

National Data Archive on Child Abuse and Neglect
http://www.ndacan.cornell.edu

National Dental Hygiene Certification Board
http://www.ndhcb.ca

Northeast Regional Board of Dental Examiners,
Inc. (NERB)
http://www.nerb.org

Occupational Safety and Health Administration
http://www.osha.gov

Prevent Child Abuse America (U.S. Department of Health and Human Services: Administration for Children and Families)
http://www.childabuse.org

Southern Regional Testing Agency, Inc, (SRTA)
http://www.srta.org

U.S. Census Bureau
http://www.census.gov

U.S. Department of Labor, OSHA Workers' Page
http://www.osha.gov/as/opa/worker/index.html

Violence in the Workplace
http://www.cdc.gov/niosh/violcont.html

Violence in the Workplace
http://www.cdc.gov/niosh/injury/traumaviolence.html

Violence in the Workplace
http://www.cdc.gov/niosh/violfs.html

Violence in the Workplace
http://www.cdc.gov/niosh/2002—101.html

WebMD
http://www.webmd.com

Western Regional Testing Agency, Inc (WREB)
http://wreb.org

Win-win Negotiation, Mind Tools
http://www.mindtools.com/CommSkll/NegotiationSkills.htm

Note: Internet sites may change. Searching the Internet via key words is another option for obtaining information.

GLOSSARY

Abandon: to end a patient–provider relationship; terminate treatment or refrain from seeing the patient.

Access to care: individual's ability to obtain timely personal health (and dental) care; access to care is hindered by financial resources, location of providers, distance and transportation problems, and sociological barriers.

Accounts receivable: accounts, usually incurred by patients, whereby the money is owed to the practice for services received.

Accreditation: process by which standards are guaranteed.

Act utilitarian: a utilitarian who is concerned with individual acts.

Advanced appointment system: a system that allows the patient to obtain an appointment in the distant future, for example, 3 months or 6 months.

Advanced dental therapist: a provider who can administer a wide range of clinical services, including basic restorative services and extractions, and who could administer care without a dentist on site.

Advocacy: act of directly representing or defending others; lobbying is social advocacy or political advocacy.

Assault: threatening to harm an individual; a type of tort or civil wrong. Technical assault is no intention of harming; similar to technical battery.

Assent: permission granted by a minor or another person who is unable to give consent.

Authoritative management: occurs when the dentist or one person makes all the decisions for the practice.

Autonomy: self-determination; a core value or ethical principle found in a code of ethics; necessary for informed consent and patient as partner in treatment.

Battery: touching an individual with the intention to harm; a type of tort or civil wrong. Technical battery is with no intention of harming but actually touching without permission; similar to technical assault.

Beneficence: doing what will benefit the patient; a core value or ethical principle found in a code of ethics.

Benefits: anything over and above salary and provided by the employer at no cost to the employee.

Capitation: a flat fee provided to a dentist or provider by a third party or insurance payor regardless of the dental procedures performed based on the number of consumers enrolled on the plan.

Case law: common law; law determined by court judgments, not by legislation.

Cash flow: a steady flow of revenue or income for services provided.

Certification: recognition of advanced training granted by a nongovernmental entity; not to be confused with a license granted by government.

Child abuse: any act that endangers or impairs a child's physical or emotional health or development.

Civil law: one of two types of statutory law; concerns offenses or wrongful acts against an individual person, property, or reputation; includes tort and contract law; seeks to compensate the victim.

Collaborative practice: A collaborative practice dental hygienist may be employed or engaged by a health care facility or nonprofit entity to provide complete dental hygiene scope of practice care under general supervision to persons who have difficulty accessing oral health care services.

Common law: case law; law determined by court judgments, not by legislation.

Compounding interest: interest paid on both the principal and the accumulated interest.

Confidentiality: avoidance of disseminating or revealing any personal or private information about the patient; a core value or ethical principle found in a code of ethics; also, duty to the patient bound by law.

Consequentialist theory: type of normative ethics that judges an action as right or wrong by the consequences; utilitarianism is the best-known consequentialist theory.

Contracts: legal agreements; part of civil law; can be either implied or expressed.

Contributory negligence: actions or behaviors of a patient that contribute to the patient's own harm.

Cost of living: an index that correlates with increases in standards of living. How much does it cost to maintain a standard of life? Increases may range from 3% to 5% each year based on increases for all products purchased by consumers.

Credentials: qualifications that entitle an individual to license, authority, and so on.

Criminal law: one of two types of statutory law; concerns offenses against society; seeks to punish the offender through loss of life or liberty or through fines.

Cross training: implies that each member in the office has been trained to perform duties of other staff members; limitations will apply for licensed personnel.

Culture: prevailing beliefs, customs, values, and rituals shared by a specific group of people (or a society).

Decision making: process using critical thinking skills to arrive at a judgment or conclusion.

Defamation: making false statements that harms an individual's reputation; can be either libel (written) or slander (oral); involves communication to a third person; a type of tort or civil wrong.

Dental health aide therapist: trained health care professionals who provide oral exams, preventive dental services, simple restorations, stainless steel crowns, extractions and X-rays in the rural territories of Alaska.

Dental health maintenance organization: an organization designed to promote the prevention of oral disease by enabling consumers to enroll for an annual fee and then to have access to all procedures without having to pay an additional fee.

Dental hygiene diagnosis: the act of identifying an actual or potential human need deficit related to oral health or disease that the dental hygienist is educated and licensed to treat.

Dental therapist: is a licensed dental auxiliary who specializes in treating children's teeth and oral hygiene.

Deontology: branch of normative ethics that emphasizes duties.

Dilemma: situation necessitating a choice between two equal, especially undesirable, alternatives.

Direct approach: a system where staff members of the dental office will directly contact patients to schedule periodic examination and dental hygiene appointments.

Disability: any physical, condition, injury or illness that disables a person to perform duties that are employment related in a normal fashion.

Disparities: inequalities between groups.

Distributive justice: fair distribution or allocation of resources.

Domestic violence: violence that occurs in the home or within the family; spouse abuse, wife battering, or abusing an individual having an intimate contact.

Duty: obligation; action that ought to be done regardless of consequences.

Efficacy: to produce effects or intended results.

Elderly abuse: physical or sexual abuse, emotional confinement, passive neglect, willful deprivation, and financial exploitation.

Ethical dilemma: conflict between moral obligations that are difficult to reconcile.

Ethics: discipline consisting of thoughts and ideas about morality; judging actions right or wrong.

Evaluations: review of employee performance based on job descriptions and/or determination of the worth or value of an employee by an employer or a supervisor.

Fidelity: faithful to promises and obligations; a core value or ethical principle found in a code of ethics; closely related to veracity, trust, and confidentiality.

Forensic dentistry: dental specialty that uses evidence such as bite marks, human teeth, and dental records to identify human remains, assess injuries, and provide other facts or data in criminal or civil cases.

Free-rein management: occurs when no one particular person is the authority figure in the practice.

Health maintenance organization (HMO): managed care; system of health care delivery that controls utilization and costs of service to deliver cost-effective care.

HIPAA: acronym for Health Insurance Portability and Accountability Act of 1996, passed by the U.S. Congress to guarantee continuity of health insurance, maintain confidentiality of electronic records, and protect the privacy of written and oral information.

Huddle: a daily meeting that occurs each morning or other agreed-on time wherein the entire staff reviews the daily schedule and patient charts.

Independent practice: a dental hygiene practice separate or independent from a dental practice.

Indirect approach: a system that uses other methods of contacting patients for future appointments: postcards, mailers, and notices.

Informed consent: patient's acceptance (or refusal) of a line of treatment based on the information provided by a health care provider; an ethical and legal consideration.

Insurance fraud: a criminal act which is intentional or deliberate misrepresentation for financial or personal gain.

Jurisprudence: science or philosophy of law.

Justice: fairness and impartiality; a core value or ethical principle found in a code of ethics.

Liability: the state of being liable to another party (providing a service that has been promised).

Libel: written or published defamation; one of two types of defamation, the other being slander (oral).

Life insurance: insurance in which a stipulated sum of money is paid to a named beneficiary or beneficiaries at the death of the insured.

Lobbying: social advocacy or political advocacy to influence a legislator.

Mail system: a system that uses regular mail delivery to notify consumers of a needed dental visit. Postcards are typically used, and the patient becomes responsible to follow through with obtaining the appointment.

Malpractice: professional negligence; not performing standard of care and harm results; part of tort law, civil law.

Managed care: health maintenance organization (HMO); system of health care delivery that controls utilization and costs of service to deliver cost-effective care.

Marketing: a social and managerial process by which individuals and groups obtain what they need through exchange of products or services that have value.

Medicaid: federal government health care assistance, enacted by each state, for indigent or low-income individuals.

Medicare: In the United States, federal government health care assistance for individuals 65 years or older; largest health insurance program in United States. In Canada, universal health insurance under the Canada Health Act.

Merit: recognition of worth or value.

Mid-level practitioner: a mid-level provider can do simple invasive procedures done only by dentists.

Negligence: not performing or measuring up to the standards of a reasonable and prudent person and harm results; see *malpractice* and *professional negligence*.

Net worth: the amount of money remaining after all debts are paid.

Nonmaleficence: to do no harm to others; a core value or ethical principle found in a code of ethics.

Normative ethics: metaethics; branch of ethics that recommends specific actions as right and justified.

Online trading: the act of investing, buying, or selling stocks, mutuals funds, or notes using an Internet source.

Overhead: the amount (in money or finances) that it costs to operate a business.

Parentalism: paternalism; acting like a father or parent who knows what is best for the patient; making a decision for the patient.

Participatory management: occurs when all staff members participate in the decision-making process for the practice.

Paternalism: parentalism; acting like a father or parent who knows what is best for the patient; making a decision for the patient.

Patients' bill of rights: rights of a patient guaranteed by the provider, the institution providing services, or the government; duties of the provider the patient can expect.

Policy manuals: each practice will develop manuals that assist all personnel in understanding the rules, regulations, and duties that pertain to the daily operations of the practice; manuals can be developed for numerous categories.

Portfolio: a collection of papers, manuscripts, drawings; anything pertinent to a specific assignment, job, or class.

Preauthorization: the submission of a dental insurance claim requesting permission and/or allowed monies designated for specific procedures prior to the actual delivery of the procedure.

Preceptorship: entails training on the job, by an employer, then receiving licensure after passing a written test.

Preferred provider organization: an organization where a dentist or provider agrees to provide dental care to patients enrolled in the plan at discounted fees; in return, the dentist or provider is given access to a pool of patients who have the dental coverage.

Prima facie: at first sight; moral obligation that appears at first sight as compelling but may be overridden by stronger duties.

Privilege: valid claim earned by effort and hard work.

Production: the total amount or costs of services given to patients; production can be calculated by the day, week, month, or year.

Professional negligence: malpractice; not performing standard of care and harm results; part of tort law, civil law.

Public relations: the promotion and protection of a company's image.

Registered dental hygienist in alternative practice: after additional education and licensure RDHAPSs may practice unsupervised in homes, schools, residential facilities, and other institutions, and in Dental Health Professional Shortage Areas.

Résumé: a summary of facts about one's education, employment, memberships, and qualifications.

Rights: valid claims guaranteed in a society.

Risk management: term used to describe the actions taken to prevent financial loss or possible legal action.

Rule utilitarian: a utilitarian who is concerned with the rule from which an action is derived.

Scope of practice: functions that a professional or licensed practitioner is allowed to perform.

Self-regulation: profession oversees (i.e., regulates or licenses) its own members; profession not being regulated by another profession.

Sexual harassment: unwelcomed or unwanted behaviour or activities of a sexual nature that occurs between two or more individuals of unequal power.

Slander: oral or spoken defamation; one of two types of defamation, the other being libel (written).

Spouse abuse: domestic violence; battered wife; control over an individual with whom one is intimate.

Standard negligence: ordinary negligence; negligence that does not involve patient care or professional responsibilities.

Standard of care: minimal level of care that is recognized by a professional group as appropriate.

State assistance: a state-funded program for qualified consumers that will allow health and dental care delivery at no cost to the consumer.

Statutory law: law enacted by legislation; two types of statutory law are criminal law and civil law.

Surrogate: legal representative for a patient who is a minor or an incompetent.

Team concept: the idea that all members act as part of a team and work to attain a common goal.

Technical assault: touching without permission but with no intention of harming; similar to technical battery.

Technical battery: touching without permission but with no intention of harming; similar to technical assault.

Teleology: consequentialism; branch of normative ethics that emphasizes consequences of an action.

Torts: civil wrongs; can be intentional or unintentional; part of civil law.

Trust: confidence in the truth or action; a core value or ethical principle found in a code of ethics.

Unsupervised practice: Unsupervised dental hygiene may be performed by licensed dentists and licensed dental hygienists without the supervision of a licensed dentist.

Usual, customary, and reasonable: refers to the fees a dentist will charge for the services offered to consumers.

Utility: usefulness of an action; underlies the theory of utilitarianism.

Veracity: telling the truth; a core value or ethical principle found in a code of ethics.

Virtue ethics: type of ethics that places emphasis on character traits of the person rather than the behavior.

WORKS CITED

American Dental Association. (1998). *Proceedings: Dentists C.A.R.E. Conference*. Chicago: Author.

American Dental Association. (2004). *Dental education at a glance*. Washington, DC: Author.

American Dental Association. (2010). *2008–2009 survey of dental education: Academic programs, enrollment, and graduates* (vol. 1). Washington, DC: Author

American Dental Association. (no date). *Medicare will not pay for most dental care & dentures*. Chicago: Author. Retrieved July 11, 2010.

American Dental Education Association. (2003). *Competencies for entry into the profession of dental hygiene*. Washington, DC: Author.

American Dental Education Association. (2009). *Statement on professionalism in dental education*. Washington, DC: Author.

American Dental Hygienists' Association, Division of Governmental Affairs (1996). Stateline. *Access, 10*(10), 38–39.

American Dental Hygienists' Association. (1999). *Bylaws and code of ethics*. Chicago: Author.

American Dental Hygienists' Association, Division of Governmental Affairs (2004). Stateline special: Less restrictive supervision practice makes strides. *Access, 18*(10), 47–49.

American Dental Hygienists' Association. (2005). Press room: *Advance dental hygiene practitioner frequently asked questions*. http:www.adha.org/media/bacground/adhp.htm

American Dental Hygienists' Association. (2005). Press room: *ADHA's response to ADA study: The economic impact of unsupervised dental hygiene practice and its impact on access to care in the state of Colorado*. http:www.adha.org

American Dental Hygienists' Association. (2009). Survey of dental hygienists in the United States, 2007: Executive summary. Chicago, IL: Author

Ashur, M. S. (1993). Community oriented primary care approach to domestic violence. *Journal of the American Medical Association, 296*(18), 2367.

Astroth, D.B., & Cross-Oline, G.N., (1998). Pilot study of six Colorado dental hygiene independent practices. *Journal of Dental Hygiene, 72*(1):13–22.

Barker, R. L. (2003). *The social work dictionary*. (5th ed.). Washington, DC: National Association of Social Workers Press

Babinski, D. (1999). Bridge Network, Inc. Dental Products and Services. http:www.bridge-network.com

Bebeau, M. J., Rest, J. R., & Yamoor, C. M. (1985). Measuring dental students' ethical sensitivity. *Journal of Dental Education, 49*(4), 225–235.

Bergmann, T. (2000). The beauty of managed care. *RDH*, 20(6), 46–45, 100.

Berry, J. (2005). Unsupervised hygiene practice not improving access to dental care in Colorado, study shows *Journal of the American Dental Association,* 136, 289.

Bressman, J. K. (1993). Risk management for the '90s. *Journal of the American Dental Association, 124*(3), 63–67.

Board of Dental Examiners of Alabama. (2009). *Alabama dental hygiene program: Dentist-instructor manual*. Hoover, AL: Author.

Cady, C. (2009). Sued over caries? *Modern Hygienist, 5*(3), 22–23.

Canadian Dental Hygienists Association. (2002). *Code of ethics*. Ottawa: Author.

Canadian Dental Hygienists Association. (2010, June). *CDHA congratulates Newfoundland and Labrador dental hygienists on self regulation*. Ottawa: Author.

Canadian Dental Hygienists Association. (no date). *Client's bill of rights*. http:www.cda.ca

Carranza, F. A., & Perry, D. (1996). *Clinical periodontology for the dental hygienist.* Philadelphia: Saunders.

Chapdelaine, A., Ruiz, A., Warchal, J., & Wells, C. (2005). Service-learning code of ethics. Bolton, MA: Anker.

Center for Health Workforce Studies. (2004). *The professional practice environment of dental hygienists in the fifty states and the District of Columbia, 2001.* Albany: University of Albany of the State University of New York. http://bhpr.hrsa.gov/healthworkforce/reports/hygienists/dh1.htm

Centers for Disease Control. (1991). Recommendations for preventing transmission of human immunodeficiency virus and hepatitis B virus to patients during exposure-prone invasive procedures. *Morbidity and Mortality Weekly Report, 40* (No. RR-8, July 12), 1–9.

Centers for Disease Control. (1997). IIOSH Facts: Violence in the workplace. http:www.cdc.gov/niosh/violfs.html

Centers for Disease Control. (1998). Are patients in a dentist's or doctor's office at risk of getting HIV? Retrieved October 1, 2001, from http:www.cdc.gov/hiv/pubs/faq/faq29.htm

Centers for Disease Control. (2003). Guidelines for infection control in dental health care settings. *Morbidity and Mortality Weekly Report, 52* (No. RR-17, December 19), 1–61.

Cobban, S. J., Wilson, M. P., Covington, P. A., Miller, B., Moore, D. P., & Rudin, S. L. (2005). Dental hygiene student experience with ethically problematic situations. *Canadian Journal of Dental Hygiene 39*(2), 67–74.

Commission on Dental Accreditation (1998). *Accreditation standards for dental hygiene programs.* Chicago: American Dental Association.

Commission on Dental Accreditation (2007). *Accreditation standards for dental hygiene programs.* Chicago: American Dental Association.

Community—Campus Partnership for Health. (2004). *Service-learning.* Retrieved August 31, 2004, from http://depts.washington.edu/ccph/servicelearningsres.html

Coughlin, S. S. (2009). Ethics in epidemiology and public health practice (2nd ed.). Washington, DC: American Public Health Association.

Covey, S. (1990). *The 7 habits of highly effective people: Restoring the character ethic.* New York: Simon & Schuster.

Curley, A. W. (1997). Malpractice: The dentist's perspective. *Journal of the American College of Dentists, 64*(2), 21–24.

Curran, A. E., & Darby, M. (1990). Dental hygiene preceptorship: An issue of risk management. *Journal of Dental Hygiene, 64*(7), 290–295.

da Fonseca, M. A., & Idelberg, J. (1993). The important role of dental hygienists in the identification of child maltreatment. *Journal of Dental Hygiene, 67*(3), 135–139.

Daniel, S. J., & Harfst, S. A. (2002). *Mosby's dental hygiene: Concepts, cases and competencies.* St. Louis, MO: Mosby.

Daniel, S. J., Harfst, S. A., & Wilder, R. S. (2008). *Mosby's dental hygiene: Concepts, cases and competencies* (2nd ed.). St. Louis, MO: Mosby.

Darby, M. L. (Ed.). (1998). *Comprehensive review of dental hygiene* (4th ed.). St. Louis, MO: Mosby.

Darby, M., & Walsh, M. (2003). *Dental hygiene theory and practice* (2nd ed.). St. Louis, MO: Saunders.

Darby, M. L, & Walsh, M. M. (2010). *Dental hygiene theory and practice* (3rd ed.). St. Louis, MO: Saunders.

Davison, J. A. (2000). *Legal and ethical considerations for dental hygienists and assistants.* St. Louis, MO: Mosby.

Dental Products Report. (March 2001). Image Management Software. http:www.televere.com; http:www.dentalproducts.net/index.

DesAutels, P., Battin, M., & May, L. (1999). *Praying for a cure: When medical and religious practices conflict.* Lanham, MD: Rowman & Littlefield.

DeVore, C. (1997). Legal risk management for the dental hygienist. *Journal of Practical Hygiene, 6*(4), 59–61.

Dietz, E. (2000). *Dental office management.* Albany, NY: Delmar.

Duley, S. I., Fitzpatrick, P. G., Zornosa, X., Lambert, C. A., & Mitchell, A. (2009). Dental hygiene students' attitudes toward ethical dilemmas in practice. *Journal of Dental Education, 73*(3), 345–357.

Edelman, M. A., & Menz, B. L. (1996). Selected comparisons and implications of a national rural and urban survey in health care access, demographics, and policy issues. *Journal of Rural Health, 12*(3), 197–205.

Edgington, E. M., Pimlott, J. F. L., & Cobban, S. J. (2009). Societal conditions driving the need for advocacy education in dental hygiene. *Canadian Journal of Dental Hygiene, 43*(6), 274–276.

Elderly Abuse and Neglect Program. (1991). *Elderly abuse awareness.* Springfield: Illinois Department on Aging.

Emmot, L. (1999). Boys & toys. *RDH*, October, 81–86.

Ferguson, D. A., Sweet, D. J., & Craig, B. J. (2008). Forensic dentistry and dental hygiene: How can the dental hygienist contribute? *Canadian Journal of Dental Hygiene 42(4), 203–211.*

Fernandes, V. A. (2009). An international dental hygienist in America. *Access, 23*(8), 16, 33.

Fitch, P. (2004). Cultural competence and dental hygiene care delivery: Integrating cultural care into the dental hygiene process of care. *Journal of Dental Hygiene,* 78(1), 11–29.

Ganssle, C. L. (1995). *Managing oral healthcare delivery: A resource for dental professionals.* Albany, NY: Delmar.

Garvin, C., & Siedge, S. H. (1992). Sexual harassment within dental offices in Washington state. *Journal of Dental Hygiene, 66*(4), 178–184.

Geurink, K. V. (2005). *Community oral practice for the dental hygienists.* (2nd ed.). St. Louis, MO: Elsevier Saunders.

Gibson-Howell, J. C. (1996). Domestic violence identification and referral. *Journal of Dental Hygiene, 70*(2), 74–77.

Gibson-Howell, J. C. , Gladwin, M. A., Hicks, M. J., Tudor, J.F.E., & Rashid, R. G. (2008). Instruction in dental curricula to identify and assist domestic violence victims. *Journal of Dental Education, 72*(11), 1277–1289.

Givens, A.T. (2009). Dental hygiene: One profession, one license, one national clinical examination. *Access, 23*(8), 16.

Glantz, L., Mariner, W., & Annas, G. (1992). Risky business: Setting public health policy for HIV-infected health care professionals. *Milbank Quarterly, 70*(1), 43–79.

Gutheil, T., & Appelbaum, P. (1982). *Clinical handbook of psychiatry and the law.* New York: McGraw-Hill.

Gutheil, T., & Appelbaum, P. (2000). *Clinical handbook of psychiatry and the law.* (3rd ed.). Philadelphia: Lippincott, Williams & Wilkins.

Gutkowski, S. (2003). Who's talking? *RDH, 23*(4), 40, 93.

Hanks, P. (Ed.). (1986). *The Collins English dictionary.* (2nd ed.). London: William Collins Sons.

Haring, J. I., & Jansen, L. (2000). *Dental radiography: Principles and techniques.* (2nd ed.). Philadelphia: Saunders.

Having, K., Davis, J., Lautar, C., & Woodward, B. (2010). Assessment of healthcare faculty interest in Internet-based international education collaboration and exchange. *International Electronic Journal of Health Education.*13, 111–124.

Having, K., & Lautar, C. (2008). Cultural competency and healthcare education. *Academic Exchange Quarterly, 12*(2), 227–231.

Hazel, C. (1998). The vital role of practice marketing. *Hycomb Marketing Tools for Dentists.* http:www.hycomb.com

Health Canada. (2002). Commission on the future of health care in Canada. Retrieved December 31, 2004, from http:www.hc-sc.gc.ca/english/care/romanow/hcc0403.html

Healthcare Providers Service Organization. (2004). Unanticipated outcomes must be disclosed. *HIPSO Risk Advisor*, 7, 4–5.

Herren, M. C., & Bryon, R. J. (2005). Elder abuse update. *General Dentistry, 53*(3), 217–219.

Honderich, T. (Ed.). (1995). *The Oxford companion to philosophy*. New York: Oxford University Press.

Hood, C. A., Hope, T., & Dove, P. (1998). Videos, photographs, and patient consent. *British Medical Journal*, 316, 1009–1011. Retrieved May 22, 2005, from http://bmj.bmjjournals. com/cgi/content/full/316/7136/1009

Illinois Department on Aging. (1999). *Elderly abuse. . . . It happens.* Springfield: State of Illinois.

Illinois Department of Human Rights. (2010). Illinois Human Rights Act, PA 96–574. Springfield, IL: Illinois General Assembly. www.state.il.us/dhr/rule.

Illinois Department of Financial and Professional Regulation. (2006). *Dental hygiene licensure package.* Springfield, IL: State of Illinois. www.idfpr.org.

Illinois Department of Professional Regulation. (2004). *Rules for the administration of the Illinois Dental Practice Act.* Springfield: State of Illinois.

International Federation of Dental Hygiene. (2003). Code of Ethics. Victoria, Australia: Author. www.idhf.org.

Jaeks, K. S. (2008, June). Speaking out loud. *RDH*, 74–76, 78, 80, 116.

Jesse, J., Desai, S., & Oshita, P. (2004). *The evolution of lasers in dentistry: Ruby to YSGG. Dental Economics*, July.

Johnson, B. (2006). *Active shooter: Protecting the lives of innocents in shooting situations.* Nashville, TN: Regional Organizes Crime Information Center.

Johnson, P. M. (2009). International profiles of dental hygiene 1987to 2006: A 31-nation comparative study. *International Dental Journal, 59*(3), 63–77.

Johnson, O. N., McNally, M. A., & Essay, C. E. (1999). *Essentials of dental radiography for dental assistants and hygienists* (6th ed.). Stamford, CT: Appleton & Lange.

Kessler, H., Bick, J., Pottage, J., & Benson, C. (1992). AIDS: Part 1. *Disease-a-Month, 38*(9), 633–639.

Knapp, K. K., & Hardwick, K. (2000). The availability and distribution of dentists in rural zip codes and primary care health professional shortage areas (PC-HPSA) zip codes: Comparison with primary care providers. *Journal of Public Health Dentistry, 60*(1), 43–48.

Knight, R. (2010, February 3). Dealing with sexual harassment in the operatory. *Dental Products Report.* http//:www.dentalproductsreport.com

Knowles, R., & Nocera, J. (2009). Integrating political advocacy into the dental hygiene classroom. *Access, 23*(6), 16–17.

Kohlberg, L. A. (1967). Moral and religious education and the public school: A developmental view. In T. Sizer (Ed.), *Religion and public education* (pp. 164–183). Boston: Houghton Mifflin.

Kotler, P. (1997). *Marketing management: Analysis, planning, implementation and control.* (9th ed.). Upper Saddle River, NJ: Prentice Hall.

Lautar, C. (1995). Is dental hygiene a profession? A literature review. *Probe, 29*(4), 127–132.

LeBlanc, H. P., Nawrot, R., Bernstein, F., Mumford, S., Lautar, C., & Beaver, S. (1997). *Southern seven oral health needs assessment.* Unpublished manuscript.

Lloyd, P. (2010). Traveling the world. *Northwest Dentistry Journal.* Minnesota Dental Association. http://www.mndental.org/features/ 2009/02/02/95

Litch, C. S., & Liggett, M. L. (1992). Consent for dental therapy in severely ill patients. *Journal of Dental Education, 56*(5), 298–311.

Liu, J., Probst, J. C., Martin, A. B., Wang, J. Y., & Salinas, C. F. (2007). Disparities in dental insurance coverage and dental care among U. S. children: The National Survey of Children's Health. *Pediatrics, 119*(Suppl. 1), S12–21.

Loesche, W. L. (1997). Association of the oral flora with important medical diseases. *Current Opinion in Periodontology, 4*, 21–28.

Lopez, N., Wadenya, R., & Berthold, P. (2003). Effective recruitment and retention strategies for underrepresented minority students: Perspectives from dental students. *Journal of Dental Education, 67*(10), 1107–1112.

Lux, J. A., & Lavigne, S. E. (2004). Your mouth: Portal to your body. *Probe, 38*(4), 155–171.

Masek, R. T. (1999). Cutting time and expenses with the Cerec 2 CAD/CAM system. *Dentistry Today, 18*(4), 64–68.

McKee, L. (2000). Workplace issues. *Access, 14*(6), 16–24.

McPhaul, K. M., & Lipscomb, J. A. (2004). Workplace violence in health care: Recognized but not regulated. *Online Journal of Issues in Nursing, 9*(3), Manuscript 6, www.nursing-world.org

Metropolitan State University, St. Paul. (2009). Master of science oral health care practitioner. Retrieved April 3, 2010, from http://www.met-rostate.edu.

Meyer, M. J., & Schiff, M. (2004). *HIPAA: The questions you didn't know to ask.* Upper Saddle River, NJ: Pearson Prentice Hall.

Miles, L. (1999). CEO practice management consultant. http://lindamiles.worldnet.att.net

Miller, R. D. (2006). *Problems in health care law.* (9th ed.). Boston: Jones & Bartlett.

Miller, R. D., & Hutton, R. C. (2000). *Problems in health care law* (8th ed.). Gaithersburg, MD: Aspen.

Monagle, J. F., & Thomasma, D.C. (2002). *Health care ethics: Critical issues for the 21st century.* Boston: Jones and Bartlett.

Mueller-Joseph, L., & Peterson, M. (1995). *Dental hygiene process: Diagnosis and care planning.* Albany, NY: Delmar.

Munson, R. (1996). *Interventions and reflection: Basic issues in medical ethics.* (5th ed.). Belmont, CA: Wadsworth.

Murphree, K. R., Campbell, P. R., Gutmann, M. E., Plichta, S. B., Nunn, M. E., McCann, A. L., & Gibson, G. (2002). How well prepared are Texas dental hygienists to recognize and report elderly abuse? *Journal of Dental Education, 66*(11), 1274–1280.

Nash, D. (2004). Developing a pediatric oral health therapist to help address oral health disparities among children. *Journal of Dental Education, 68*(1), 8–20.

Nathe, C. N. (2005). *Dental public health: Contemporary practice for the dental hygienist* (2nd ed.). Upper Saddle River, NJ: Pearson Education.

National Cancer Institute. (no date). If you have cancer and have Medicare: You should know about clinical trails. Retrieved July 4, 2010, from *http://www.cancer.gov/clinicltrails/resources/medicare-and-cancer-trails.*

National Institutes of Health. (1979). *The Belmont report: Ethical principles and guidelines for the protection of human subjects of research.* Retrieved May 31, 2005, from http://ohrs.od.nih.gov/guidelines/Belmont.html

Nelms, A. P., Gutmann, M. E., Solomon, E. S., DeWald, J. P., & Campbell, P. R. (2009). What victims of domestic violence need from the dental profession. Journal of Dental Education, 73(4), 490–498.

Neiburger, E. J. (1998). How to profit from computers: 10 rules for selecting a computer system. *Dental Economics*, August, 96–99.

Neish, N., & MacDonald, L. (2003). CDHA Code of Ethics Workshop: Application to day-to-day work. *Probe, 37*(1), 27–33.

Nelson, D. M. (2000). *Review of dental hygiene.* Philadelphia: Saunders.

New Mexico Dental Hygienists' Association. (2010). About collaborative practice. Retrieved April 13, 2010,from http://nmdha.org/legislative/state-articel3.php

New York Life. (2010). Whole life insurance. *New York Life Insurance Company.* Retrieved February 14, 2010, from *http://www.newyorklife.com/nyl/v/index*

Newell, K. J., Young, L. J., & Yamoor, C. M. (1985). Moral reasoning in dental hygiene students. *Journal of Dental Education, 49*(2), 79–84.

Newman, J. F., & Gift, H. C. (1992). Regular pattern of preventive dental services—A measure of access. *Social Science and Medicine, 35*(8), 997–1001.

Nierenberg, J. (1999). *Women and the art of negotiation*. New York: The Negotiation Institute. http:www.negotiation.com

Northouse, P. (2007). *Leadership theory and practice* (4th ed). Thousand Oaks, CA: Sage.

Ohio State Dental Board. (2000). *Ohio State Dental Board law and rules*. Columbus: State of Ohio.

Oldenquist, A. G. (1978). *Moral development: Text and readings*. (2nd ed.). Boston: Houghton Mifflin.

Oral, R. (2004). Denial of critical care/child neglect. *EPSDT Care for Kids Newsletter*. Iowa City: University of Iowa Retrieved from http//:www.iowaepsdt.org

Ozar, D. T., & Sokol, D. J. (1994). *Dental ethics at chairside: Professional principles and practical applications*. St. Louis, MO: Mosby.

Paige, B. E. (1977). Malpractice: An overview for the dental hygienist. *Dental Hygiene, 51*(4), 167–173.

Palmer. P. R. (2002). Access extra. *Access, 16*(9), 16, 18.

Patients' Bill of Rights Act. (1999). U.S. Congress (July 8). Washington, DC: U.S. Government Printing Office.

Patton, L. L., White, R. A., & Field, M. J. (2001). Extending Medicare coverage to medically necessary dental care. *Journal of the American Dental Association, 132*(9), 1294–1299.

Peck, S. B. (2000). Testimony before the House Appropriations Subcommittee on Labor, Health and Human Services, Education and Related Agencies on fiscal year 2001 appropriations. *Access, 14*(6), 41–43.

Pennington, A., Darby, M., Bauman, D., Plichta, S., & Schnuth, ML. (2000). *Journal of Dental Hygiene, 74*(4), 288–95.

Pollack, B. R., & Marinelli, R. (1988). Ethical, moral and legal dilemmas in dentistry: The process of informed decision making. *Journal of Law and Ethics in Dentistry, 1*(1), 27–36.

Pozgar, G. D. (2004). *Legal aspects of health care administration*. (9th ed.). Boston: Jones and Bartlett.

Public Health Agency of Canada. (1998). Infected health care worker: risk of transmission of bloodborne pathogens. Retrieved December 31, 2004, from http:www/phac-aspc.gc.ca/publicat/info/infbbp_e.html

Public Health Futures Illinois. (2000). *Illinois plan for public health systems change*. Springfield: State of Illinois.

Purtilo, R. (1999). *Ethical dimensions in the health professions*. (3rd ed.). Philadelphia: Saunders.

Rawls, J. (1971). *A theory of justice*. Cambridge, MA: Belknap Press of Harvard University Press.

Reis-Schmidt, T. (1998). Trends in dentistry. *Dental Products Report*, August, 24–31.

Rest, J. R. (1986). *Moral development: Advances in research and theory*. New York: Praeger.

Reynolds, R. (2004). HIPAA: Continuing education course. *Journal of Dental Hygiene, 78*(3). Electronic reprint generated by Ingenta, http:www.ingenta.com

Rich, J. M., & DeVitis, J. L. (1985). *Theories of moral development*. Springfield, IL: Charles C. Thomas.

Richardson, F. (2004). The Canadian view of self-regulation. *RDH, 24(3)*, 18–21.

Richardson, F. (2005). Power, control, and economics: A case study in professional ethics. *Canadian Journal of Dental Hygiene*, 39(3), 97–102.

Ring, T. (2003). HIPAA and its implications for dental hygiene. *Access, 17*(4), 20–28.

Ring, T. (2004). The advanced dental hygiene practitioner. *Access, 18*(8), 14–20.

Rosoff, A. (1981). *Informed consent: A guide for health care providers*. Rockville, MD: Aspen Systems Corp.

Rost, J. (1991). *Leadership for the twenty-first century*. Westport, CT: Praeger.

Rule, J. T., & Veatch, R. M. (2004). *Ethical questions in dentistry*. (2nd ed). Chicago: Quintessence.

Saxe, M. D., & McCourt, J. W. (1991). Child abuse: A survey of ASDC members and a diagnostic-data-assessment for dentists. *Journal of Dentistry for Children, 58*(5), 361–366.

Schwimmer, A., Massoumi, M., & Barr, C. E. (1994). Efficacy of double gloving to prevent inner glove perforation during outpatient oral surgical procedures. *Journal of the American Dental Association, 125*(2), 196–198.

Scott, R. (1998). *Professional ethics: A guide for rehabilitation*. St. Louis, MO: Mosby.

Scott, R. W. (2000). *Legal aspects of documenting patient care* (2nd ed.). Gaithersburg, MD: Aspen.

Seckman, C. H. (2000). Don't call them disabled; call them practicing hygienists! *RDH, 20*(1), 34–38, 78.

Senior Health. (2004). Medicare Modernization Act of 2003. Retrieved from http://seniorhealth. about.com/od/medicare/a/medicare_drug.htm

Seifer, S. D. (1998). Service-learning: Community-campus partnerships for health professions education. *Academic Medicine, 73*(3) 273–277.

Shi, L., & Singh, D. A. (2004). *Delivering health care in America: A systems approach.* (3rd ed.). Boston: Jones and Bartlett.

Shi, L., & Singh, D. A. (2010). *Essentials of the U. S. health care system.* (2nd ed.). Boston: Jones and Bartlett.

Sohn, W., & Ismail, A. I. (2005). Regular dental visits and dental anxiety in an adult dentate population. *Journal of the American Dental Association, 136*(1), 58–66.

Sunell, S., Richardson, F., Udahl, B., Jamieson, L., & Landry, D. (2008). National competencies for dental hygiene entry-to-practice. *Canadian Journal of Dental Hygiene*, 42(1), 27–36

Stambaugh, R. V., Myers, G. C., Ebling, W. V., Beckman, B., & Stambaugh, K. A. (2000). *Endoscopic visualization of submarginal gingival root surfaces*. Paper presented at IADR 2000, Washington, DC.

State Farm Life Insurance Company (2010). Term life insurance. Retrieved February 14, 2010, from http://www.statefarm.com/insurance/ life_annuity/life/term/term.asp

Stern, J. (2003). *A study of decision-making strategies for resolving common ethical dilemmas by fourth year dental students*. Unpublished master's thesis, Concordia University, Montreal.

Straker, D. (2009). Leadership vs. management. *Syque.com.* Retrieved on December 32, 2009, from http://www.changingminds.org.

Switankowsky, I. (1998). *A new paradigm for informed consent.* Lanham, MD: University Press of America.

The Motley Fool. (1999). Investments. http:www. netscape.com/investing

Turchetta, A. L., & Duncan, T. (2008). End the cycle of violence. *RDH, 28*(3), 44–46,48.

Turner, J., Boudreaux, M., & Lynch, V. (2009). A preliminary evaluation of health insurance coverage in the 2008 American Community Survey. Washington, DC: Department of Commerce, Economics and Statistics Administration, U. S. Census Bureau.

University of Minnesota. (2010). Dental therapist program, School of Dentistry. http:www.dentistry.umn.edu

University of the Pacific, Arthur A. Dugoni School of Dentistry. (2010). Registered dental hygienist in alternative practice (RDHAP) educational curriculum. http://www.dental.pacific.edu.

U.S. Census Bureau. (2000). *Overview of race and Hispanic origin.* Washington, DC: Department of Commerce, Economics and Statistics Administration.

U.S. Census Bureau. (2010a). *Hispanic Americans by the numbers.* Washington, DC: Department of Commerce, Economics and Statistics Administration. http://www.infoplease.com/ spot/hhmcensus1.html

U.S. Census Bureau. (2010b). Overview of race and Hispanic origin. Washington, D.C.: Department of Commerce, Economics and Statistics Administration. http://www.census.gov

U.S. Census Bureau. (2010c). *Population profile of the United States*. Washington, DC: Department of Commerce, Economics and Statistics Administration. http://www.census.gove/population/www.pop-profile/natproj.html.

U.S. Department of Health and Human Services. (2000a). *Healthy people 2010*. http:www.healthypeople.gov/gov/document

U.S. Department of Health and Human Services. (2000b). *Oral health in America: A report of the surgeon general—Executive summary*. Rockville, MD: U.S. Department of Health and Human Services, National Institute of Dental and Craniofacial Research, National Institutes of Health.

U.S. Department of Health and Human Services. (2003). *A national call to action to promote oral health*. Rockville, MD: U.S. Department of Health and Human Services, Public Health Service, Centers for Disease Control and Prevention, and National Institute of Dental and Craniofacial Research.

Department of Labor, Bureau of Labor Statistics. (2009). *Occupational outlook handbook*. http://www.bls.gov/oco/ocos097.htm

U.S. Department of Labor, Occupational Safety and Health Administration. (2005). Boodborne pathogens and needlestick prevention. Retrieved January 1, 2005, from http:www.osha.gov/SLTC/bloodbornepathogens/index.htm

Vaughn, L. D. (2007). Documentation, recordkeeping and risk management. *Access, 21*(10), 39–41.

Vaughn, L. D., & Harvey, L. (2008). The team approach to risk management. *Access*, *22*(5), 42–46.

Veal, K., Perry, M., Stavisky, J., & Herbert, K. D. (2004). The pathway to dentistry for minority students: From their perspective. *Journal of Dental Education 68*(9), 938–946.

Voelker, M. A. (2009). The dental investigation: Dental forensics and the role of the dental hygienist. *Dimensions of Dental Hygiene, 7*(10), 58–61.

Wagner, L. (1995). Bringing high technology down to earth. *Access—American Dental Hygienists Association*, April, 22–31.

Watterson, D. G. (2010, June). We're being sued. *RDH,* 52, 54, 71

Weinstein, B. D. (1993). *Dental ethics*. Philadelphia: Lea & Febiger.

Weiss, B. D. (2003). *Health literacy: A manual for clinicians*. Chicago: American Medical Association.

Wilder, R. S. (2004) The right of refusal. *Dimensions of Dental Hygiene, 2*(2), 30–31.

Wilkins, E. (2005). *Clinical practice of the dental hygienist* (9th ed.). Philadelphia: Lippincott Williams & Wilkins.

Wilkins, E. (2010). *Clinical practice of the dental hygienist* (10th ed.). Philadelphia: Lippincott Williams & Wilkins.

World Health Organization. (2003). *The world oral health report 2003: Continuous improvement of oral health in the 21st century—The approach of the WHO global Oral Health Programme*. Geneva: Author.

Wright, A. E. (2009). How are we doing? Where do we go from here? *Canadian Journal of Dental Hygiene, 43*(6), 319.

Zimmermann, K. (2004). Working: Michelle Smith, RDH. *Access, 5*(16), 12.

INDEX